The Effective Vegan Air

101 Vegan Air Fryer Recipes

By

Chef Effect

© Copyright 2017 by Chef Effect – All rights reserved.

This document is geared towards providing exact and reliable information in regards to the topic and issue covered. The publication is sold with the idea that the publisher is not required to render accounting, officially permitted, or otherwise, qualified services. If advice is necessary, legal or professional, a practiced individual in the profession should be ordered.

-From a Declaration of Principles which was accepted and approved equally by a Committee of the American Bar Association and a Committee of Publishers and Associations.

In no way is it legal to reproduce, duplicate, or transmit any part of this document in either electronic means or in printed format. Recording of this publication is strictly prohibited and any storage of this document is not allowed unless with written permission from the publisher. All rights reserved.

The information provided herein is stated to be truthful and consistent, in that any liability, in terms of inattention or otherwise, by any usage or abuse of any policies, processes, or directions contained within is the solitary and utter responsibility of the recipient reader. Under no circumstances will any legal responsibility or blame be held against the publisher for any reparation, damages, or monetary losses due to the information herein, either directly or indirectly.

Respective authors own all copyrights not held by the publisher.

The information herein is offered for informational purposes solely, and is universal as so. The presentation of the information is without contract or any type of guarantee assurance.

The trademarks that are used are without any consent, and the publication of the trademark is without permission or backing by the trademark owner. All trademarks and brands within this book, except for Chef Effect, are for clarifying purposes only and are owned by the owners themselves, not affiliated with this document.

Table of Contents

What You Need to Know About Air Frying vii

Vegan Air Frying Recipes 1

Indian and Middle Eastern Recipes 2

1. Roasted Cinnamon Sugar-Coated Chickpeas 2
2. Spicy Fried Chickpeas 3
3. Vegan Potato Cheese Balls 4
4. Air-Fried Gulab Jamun 5
5. Oil-Free Falafel 6
6. Bati Chokha 7
7. Veggie Manchurian 9
8. Crispy Healthy Veggie Rolls 10
9. Onion Pakodas 11
10. Indian Bread Rolls 12
11. Chana Dal Vada (1) 13
12. Vegan Seekh Kabab 14
13. Vegan Sabudana Vada 15
14. Hara Bhara Kabab 16
15. Curried Corn Balls 17
16. Aalu Samosa 18
17. Chakli 19
18. Chana Dal Vada (2) 20
19. Shahi Tukda 21
20. Matar Kachodi 22
21. Gujiya 23
22. Vegan-Style Pancakes 24
23. Baadal Jaam 25

Mediterranean Recipes 26

24. Asparagus-Filled Phyllo Pastry 26

25. Spanakopita Bites 27

26. Mediterranean Vegetables 28

27. Mediterranean Eggplant Chips 29

28. Mini Stuffed Grape Leaves Casserole 30

29. Air-Fried Mediterranean Yellow Squash, Zucchini and Carrots 31

30. Pesto-Potato Tofu Frittata Cups 32

31. Crispy Brussel Sprouts with Garlic 33

32. Vegan Mushroom Meatballs 34

33. Mediterranean Spiced Carrots 35

34. Greek Spinach "Meatloaf" Cups 36

35. Roasted Beets with Lemon Vinaigrette 37

36. Vegan Calzone 38

37. Best Herb Roast Potatoes 39

38. Artichoke Basil Toasts 40

39. Turmeric Roasted Cauliflower Salad with Lemon Tahini Dressing 41

40. Sautéed Carrots and Shallots with Thyme 42

41. Stuffed Mushrooms 43

Asian Recipes 44

42. Avocado Tempura 44

43. Sesame Toast 45

44. Coconut Tofu 46

45. Katsu Banh Mi 47

46. Air-Fried Tofu Scramble 49

47. Crispy Trumpet Mushroom Tempura 50

48. Spring Rolls 51

49. Fried Garlic Mushroom 52

50. Fried Tofu with Sesame-Soy Dipping Sauce 53

51. Spicy Vegan Peanut Butter Tofu with Sriracha Sauce 54

52. General Tso's Baked Cauliflower 55

53. Stick Sesame Cauliflower 56

54. Air Fried Green Beans with Garlic Sauce 57

55. Fried Ganmodoki 58

56. Vegan Katsu Curry 59

57. Crispy Kung Pao Cauliflower 61

58. Eggplant with Garlic Sauce 63

59. Asian-Style Tofu Burgers 64

60. Air-Fried Sichuan Potstickers (Gyoza) 65

American Recipes 66

61. Roasted Sweet Potatoes with Agave and Cinnamon 66

62. Apple Dumplings 67

63. Air-Fried Buffalo Cauliflower 68

64. Air-Fried Ranch Kale Chips 69

65. Texas Roadhouse Fried Pickles 70

66. Vidalia Onion Strings with Horseradish Aioli 71

67. Baked Zucchini Fries 72

68. Air-Fried Nuts 73

69. Air-Fried Banana Bread 74

70. Air-Grilled Vegan Cheese Sandwich 75

71. Broccoli Hash Brown Cheese Cups 76

72. Crispy Homemade Veggie Nuggets 77

73. Banana-Nutella Spring Rolls 78

74. Mashed Potato Tater Tots 79

75. Cheese Spinach Balls 80

76. Oil-Free French Fries 81

77. Sweet Corn Fritters 82

78. Three Sister Squash 83

79. Onion Rings 84

80. Portobello Mushroom Bacon 85

Mexican Recipes 86
   81. Quinoa Taco Meat 86
   82. Wonton Quesadillas 87
   83. Corn Tortilla Chips 88
   84. Patatas Bravas 89
   85. Air-Fried Mushroom Taquitos 90
   86. Spicy Mexican Baby Potatoes 91
   87. Air-Fried Nachos 92
   88. Mexican Plantain Chips 93
   89. Air-Fried Vegan Refried Beans 94
   90. Mexican Zucchini Burrito Boats 95
   91. Creamy Bean Taquitos 96
   92. Deep Fried Guacamole 97
   93. Baked Black Bean and Sweet Potatoes Flauta 98
   94. Crispy-Baked Tofu Tacos with Lime-Cilantro Slaw 99
   95. Baked Vegan Chimichangas 100
   96. Spicy Braised Tofu Tostadas 101
   97. Lentil Picadillo 102
   98. Vegan Chiles Rellenos 103
   99. Air-Fried Vegan Fajitas 104
   100. Crispy Black Bean Tacos 105
   101. Mexican Quinoa Stuffed Peppers 106
Conclusion 107
And Please… 107
Other Books By Chef Effect 108

What You Need to Know About Air Frying

Fried foods are the ultimate comfort foods. But with recent studies linking greasy foods to heart attacks, obesity, and diabetes, many are now staying away from enjoying them completely. However, completely avoiding fried foods can be difficult, especially if you love munching these little snacks. Now, you don't have to worry. You can always enjoy your favorite fried foods without the need to use any grease. How? Through air frying, of course!

Air frying has become the latest craze in making greasy comfort foods healthier. It is done in a kitchen appliance–an air fryer–that cooks food by circulating hot air of up to 390º Fahrenheit (200º Celsius) at high speeds around it to create a crispy layer, much as if you were cooking with oil. Health conscious people who still don't want to give up their favorite fried foods can take advantage of air fryer-ed foods.

The Benefits of Air Frying

Besides providing us comfort and satisfaction, eating fried foods provide few benefits. But with an air fryer, anyone can whip up healthy and satisfying foods minus any guilt. There are many benefits of air frying your food instead of cooking them in a conventional deep fryer. The main benefits of air frying your food is listed below:

- **Fewer calories:** Since you do not add any oil (or very little oil) to air fry your food compared to traditional frying methods, the calorie content of your meal is ultimately reduced. Remember that a cup of oil is equivalent to about 800 calories alone, so deep frying increases the caloric value of your food to a dangerously high level.
- **Easy to cook:** Never mind if you are a kitchen novice. Since air fryers are digital, they require less skill, allowing you to cook delicious dishes even if you are not good at cooking.
- **Cost effective:** Since you don't use any oil in cooking your food, you can save a lot of money from not buying cooking oil.
- **Versatile:** An air fryer is not only a fryer; you can use it to cook others types of foods too. You can use it to bake bread, make popcorn, or even make roasted vegetables.

The thing is, there are many benefits of air frying, and if you decide to make a simple change in your diet by only eating fried foods that are cooked in an air fryer, you will be able to enjoy a healthier and a more convenient life.

Best Practices When Air Frying

While it is easy to use an air fryer, using it for the first time can present some challenges. But this should not scare you from air frying your foods. After all, you get more health benefits than actually frying your food in oil. Below are the best practices and tips that you can do to successfully air fry your favorite foods.

- **Preheat the air fryer before you place your food inside:** Just like cooking in an oven, you need to preheat your air fryer so that your food will cook properly. Turn the air fryer on and preheat for at least three minutes.
- **Press the breading on your food firmly:** An air fryer has a strong fan that can blow off parts of your food. If you are putting breading on your food, make sure that you press it firmly to help it stay in place while you are cooking.
- **Use oven-safe accessories:** When cooking with an air fryer, use oven-safe accessories like small baking pans or tins where you can place your food. Oven-safe accessories can withstand extremely high temperatures, so they won't get damaged once you are cooking your food.
- **Add water to the air fryer drawer:** If you are cooking greasy foods, add water to the air fryer drawer located under the basket. This prevents the grease from getting too hot and causing it to smoke.
- **Hold your food properly:** Since air fryers have strong fans that can blow off light food particles, secure them in place using toothpicks. If food gets stuck on the fan or the heating element of the fryer, they might get burned, causing smoke to form during the cooking process.
- **Never put too many foods inside the basket:** While it is very tempting to cook a lot of food at once, overcrowding your air fryer prevents the hot air from circulating properly within the fryer, the result being that you'll end up with food that is not evenly brown or crispy.
- **Flip your food:** Halfway through the cooking time, flip your food over just as you would when cooking on a grill. This will ensure that the food will brown evenly on all sides.
- **Shake the basket:** To distribute the ingredients within the basket, you can shake the basket a few times while cooking.
- **Spray a small amount of oil:** If you are not satisfied with how brown your food is, you can spray oil halfway through the cooking process. Make sure that you spray the food lightly and not lather it with oil.

Why Embrace Veganism?

Air frying is a very healthy cooking method but you can make your life healthier if you also embrace a vegan lifestyle. Being a vegan is a lifestyle modification wherein you don't consume any types of animal products, including dairy, honey, eggs, and meat. There are countless benefits of becoming vegan but why go vegan?

To begin with, the production of animal products places a heavy toll on the environment. For instance, the grain feed used in cattle production requires tons of land and water, thus making the industry not sustainable for the planet. In addition, if you go vegan you are helping the animals by saying no to animal exploitation and cruelty. Raising livestock also results in bigger carbon emissions into the environment, because animals produce a great amount of carbon dioxide. Many advocates for this lifestyle are into recycling and have low carbon footprints because of their refusal to consume animal products.

Another reason why embracing veganism is beneficial is that it can promote health and wellness. In fact, one of the reasons why people get into veganism is for the health benefits that they can get. Scientific studies have shown that people who are on a plant-based diet have better overall health and body functions than meat eaters. Vegans get more fiber and more nutrients, as well as fewer saturated fats from eating plant-derived foods. Vegans are less prone to developing metabolic diseases like diabetes, obesity, and heart diseases.

Going vegan is really beneficial but you can make this lifestyle even more significant if you opt for more sustainable and healthy food preparation methods like air frying.

Vegan Air Frying Recipes

What makes most people scared of the vegan diet is that they think their food choices will be very limited. If you think that you can count the number of vegan air frying recipes available with your fingers, you are definitely wrong. Even if this book calls for specific vegan air frying recipes, there are hundreds of other recipes to choose from. The recipes are categorized in different cuisines so that you can easily find them within this book.

Indian and Middle Eastern Recipes

1. Roasted Cinnamon Sugar-Coated Chickpeas

Serving Size: 2

Calories: 380 per serving

Ingredients:
- 1 tbsp. sugar
- 1 tbsp. cinnamon
- 1 can chickpeas, drained and rinsed

Instructions:
1) Preheat the air fryer to 392° Fahrenheit (200° Celsius) and turn the timer to 5 minutes.
2) In a bowl, mix all the ingredients and toss until the sugar and cinnamon mixture coats the chickpeas.
3) Place the chickpeas on a small tray that fits the air fryer.
4) Once the 5 minutes is up, place the tray with the chickpeas and set the timer for 10 minutes.
5) Let the chickpeas cool inside the fryer so that they will completely dry out and will turn crunchy.

2. Spicy Fried Chickpeas

Serving Size: 3 to 4

Calories: 424 per serving

Ingredients:
- Salt to taste
- 2 15-oz. cans of chickpeas, rinsed and patted dry
- 2 tbsp. extra virgin olive oil
- 1 tsp. cinnamon
- 1 tsp. cumin
- 1 tsp. curry
- 3 tsp. cayenne pepper
- 3 tsp. smoked paprika

Instructions:
1) Preheat the air fryer to 390º Fahrenheit (199º Celsius) and set the timer for 5 minutes.
2) In a mixing bowl, combine all ingredients and toss lightly.
3) Place enough chickpeas in the fryer basket and cook for 8 to 10 minutes or until the chickpeas are crispy. Don't forget to shake the basket halfway through to cook the chickpeas evenly.
4) Once done, transfer the chickpeas to a bowl and add more seasonings as desired.

3. Vegan Potato Cheese Balls

Serving Size: 1

Calories: 520 per serving

Ingredients:
- 1 cup vegan cheese of your choice
- 1 cup bread crumbs
- A dash of salt
- 1 tsp. oregano
- 1 tsp. red chili flakes
- 3 tbsp. white flour
- 3 tbsp. corn flour
- 1 tbsp. ginger and garlic paste
- 1 tbsp. capsicum, chopped
- 1 tbsp. coriander leaves, chopped
- 3 boiled potatoes, mashed

Instructions:
1) In a mixing bowl, combine the mashed potatoes, capsicum, coriander leaves, garlic and ginger paste, 2 tbsp. of white flour, and 1 tbsp. corn flour. Mix together then add salt, oregano, chili flakes, and vegan cheese. Make small balls from the dough. Set aside.
2) In another bowl, mix 1 tbsp. of white flour and 1 tbsp. of corn flour with ½ cup water. Dip the balls in the batter, then roll them over the bread crumbs. Place the balls in the fridge for 30 minutes before cooking.
3) Preheat the air fryer to 392º Fahrenheit (200º Celsius) and set the timer for 5 minutes.
4) Air fry the balls for 10 t0 15 minutes or until golden brown.
5) Serve with chutney or tomato sauce.

4. Air-Fried Gulab Jamun

Serving Size: 2

Calories: 443 per serving

Ingredients:
- 1 cup all-purpose flour
- 1 tbsp. baking powder
- 1 cup almond milk
- 1 cup sugar
- 1 cup water

Instructions:
1) Preheat the air fryer to 356° Fahrenheit (180° Celsius) for 5 minutes.
2) Mix half a cup each of the ingredients in a mixing bowl and blend well to form a soft dough.
3) Form small balls from the dough.
4) Place the dough inside the air fryer basket and adjust the temperature to 392° Fahrenheit. Cook the dough for 10 minutes or until golden brown.
5) Serve with sugar syrup by boiling 1 cup of sugar with 1 cup of water.

5. Oil-Free Falafel

Serving Size: 2

Calories: 325 per serving

Ingredients:
- 1 cup chickpeas
- 1 tbsp. onion
- 1 tbsp. garlic
- 1 tbsp. coriander leaves
- 1 tbsp. garam masala
- 1 tsp. baking powder
- Salt to taste

Instructions:
1) In a bowl, soak the chickpeas for 12 hours until soft.
2) After 12 hours, place the chickpeas in a food processor. Add the other ingredients and pulse until smooth.
3) Coat your palm with a few drops of oil and roll small balls of the chickpea mixture.
4) Preheat the air fryer to 392º Fahrenheit (200º Celsius) for 5 minutes.
5) Place the balls inside the fryer and cook for 15 minutes.
6) Serve with chutney.

6. Bati Chokha

Serving Size: 3 to 4

Calories: 150 per serving

Ingredients:

For dough
- 1 cup wheat flour
- 1 tsp. ajwain or carom seeds
- Salt to taste
- 2 tbsp. olive oil

For stuffing
- 1 cup roasted gram flour
- 1 tbsp. green chilies
- 1 tbsp. coriander, chopped
- 1 tsp. cumin seeds, roasted
- 1 tsp. garlic, chopped
- 1 tbsp. amchur or green mango powder
- 1 tbsp. mango pickle masala
- 1 tsp. lemon juice
- 1 tbsp. onion, chopped
- 1 tsp. mustard oil
- Salt to taste

For chokha
- 2 boiled potatoes, chopped
- ½ cup tomatoes, chopped
- 1 tbsp. green chilies, chopped
- 1 tsp. onion powder
- Salt to taste

For chutney
- 1 tbsp. garlic, crushed
- 3 tomatoes, chopped
- 1 small onion, chopped
- 1 pc. red chili, chopped
- 1 tbsp. mustard seeds, crushed
- 1 tbsp. olive oil

Instructions:

1) Create the dough by sieving the flour. Add the salt, ajwain, salt, and oil. Knead the dough and add a little bit of water to create a stiff dough. Let it rest inside the fridge for 20 minutes.

2) Prepare the stuffing by mixing all the ingredients in the bowl. Add a few drops of water to make sure that the stuffing is not dry.
3) Preheat the air fryer for 5 minutes at 392° Fahrenheit (200° Celsius).
4) Make small balls from the dough and flatten them. Fill the flattened dough with the stuffing and cover the stuffing with the dough.
5) Air fry the dough for 15 minutes until golden brown.
6) Prepare the chokha by mixing the ingredients together.
7) Make the chutney by combining all ingredients in a food processor. Blend until smooth.
8) Serve the balls with chutney and chokha.

7. Veggie Manchurian

Serving Size: 2

Calories: 217 per serving

Ingredients:

For veggie balls
- 1 cup cabbage, chopped
- 1 cup carrot, chopped
- 2 tbsp. capsicum, chopped
- 1 small onion, chopped
- 2 tbsp. cornstarch
- 2 tbsp. white flour
- ½ tsp. black pepper
- Salt to taste

For Manchurian sauce
- 1 tbsp. sesame oil
- 3 cloves garlic, finely chopped
- 1 thumb-size ginger, chopped
- small chili, chopped
- 1 small onion, chopped
- tbsp. soy sauce
- ½ cup tomato sauce
- 1 tsp. red chili sauce
- 1 tsp. corn starch mixed in 3 tbsp. water
- tbsp. vinegar
- Salt and pepper to taste

Instructions:
1) Preheat the air fryer to 392º Fahrenheit (200º Celsius) for 5 minutes.
2) In a mixing bowl, mix all the ingredients together. Once incorporated, form small balls using your palms.
3) Air fry the balls for 15 minutes.
4) Meanwhile, prepare the Manchurian sauce by sautéing the garlic, ginger, chili, and onion in a skillet with sesame oil heated over medium flame. Add the rest of the ingredients. Let the sauce thicken for 3 minutes then set aside.
5) Once the balls are cooked, coat them with the Manchurian sauce.
6) Serve warm.

8. Crispy Healthy Veggie Rolls

Serving Size: 10 veggie rolls

Calories: 90 per veggie roll

Ingredients:

For dough

- 2 cups white flour
- 1 tsp. baking powder
- 1 tsp. olive oil
- 1 tsp. dried oregano
- ½ tsp. salt

For filling

- ½ cup peas
- 1 medium-sized potato, boiled and mashed
- 1 small capsicum, diced
- 1 carrot, chopped
- 1 sprig coriander, chopped
- 1 tbsp. olive oil
- ¼ cup sweet corn
- ¼ cup cabbage, chopped
- 1 small onion, chopped
- 1 clove garlic, chopped
- 1 tsp. chili powder
- 1 tbsp. chaat masala powder
- Salt to taste

Corn flour coating

- 2 tsp. corn starch
- ½ cup water
- Bread crumbs

Instructions:

1) Make the dough by mixing all ingredients in a bowl. Let the dough rest for 2 hours inside the fridge. Set aside.
2) Make the filling by heating the oil in a frying pan over medium-low heat. Add the garlic and onions and cook for a minute. Add the rest of the ingredients and add a cup of water. Let it cook and simmer until the mixture dries out.
3) Roll the dough and flatten it to make a roti.
4) Add the filling in the middle of the roti and roll it to keep the filling inside.
5) Roll in the cornstarch slurry then coat with bread crumbs.
6) Air fry in a preheated air fryer for 15 minutes at 392º Fahrenheit (200º Celsius).
7) Serve with chutney.

9. Onion Pakodas

Serving Size: 2

Calories: 210 per serving

Ingredients:
- 1 cup besan or gram flour
- 1 onion, sliced
- 1 tsp. coriander powder
- 1 tsp. carom or ajwain
- 1 tsp. cumin seed, roasted
- 1 tsp. fenugreek seeds

Instructions:
1) Preheat the air fryer to approximately 392° Fahrenheit (200° Celsius) for 5 minutes.
2) In a large bowl, mix all the ingredients together. Add a few teaspoons of water to make the pakoda moist. Do not make them too wet, otherwise the pakodas will not become crispy.
3) Form them into balls and place them in the air fryer lined with aluminum foil. Air fry for 5-10 minutes or until golden brown.

10. Indian Bread Rolls

Serving Size: 3

Calories: 230 per serving

Ingredients:
- Salt to taste
- 3 tsp. coriander leaves, chopped
- ½ tsp. chaat masala
- ¼ tsp. cumin powder
- ¼ tsp. garam masala powder
- 1 green chili, chopped
- ¼ tsp. red chili powder
- ½ tsp. black pepper, crushed
- ½ tsp. dry pomegranate seeds (crushed) or ½ tsp. dry mango powder
- 2 medium-sized potatoes, boiled and mashed
- 6 slices wheat bread

Instructions:
1) In a bowl, mix together the mashed potatoes and dry pomegranate seed powder. Add the black pepper, chili powder, green chilies, garam masala, coriander leaves, chaat masala powder, cumin, and salt. Mix everything until well combined.
2) Take a slice of bread and dampen with water. Squeeze the excess water out then place the filling in the center of the bread. Roll the bread and secure the edges with toothpick.
3) Brush the bread rolls with oil and air fry at 392° Fahrenheit (200° Celsius) in a preheated air fryer for 10 minutes or until the crust is golden brown.

11. Chana Dal Vada (1)

Serving Size: 1

Calories: 40 per serving

Ingredients:
- Salt to taste
- Oil for brushing
- A pinch of baking soda
- Half a bunch of coriander leaves
- Half a bunch of dill leaves
- Half a bunch of mint leaves
- Half a bunch of curry leaves
- 3 green chilies, chopped
- 1 small piece of ginger, chopped
- 1 small onion, chopped
- 1 tsp. rice flour
- ½ cup chana dal

Instructions:
1) Wash the chana dal and soak in ½ cup water for an hour. Drain the water in another bowl, as you will use the water for grinding later. Set aside.
2) In a food processor, add the chana dal, onion, and the different leaves. Add in salt, ginger, and chilies. Grind until a coarse paste is formed. Add a little bit of water to help through the grinding process. Add the remaining ingredients.
3) Make balls and flatten with the palm of your hand. Brush the dough with oil.
4) Cook in a 392º Fahrenheit (200º Celsius) preheated air fryer for 10 minutes or until golden brown.
5) Serve with tomato sauce or green chutney.

12. Vegan Seekh Kabab

Serving Size: 12 skewers

Calories: 40 per skewer

Ingredients:
- ½ tsp. garam masala powder
- 2 tbsp. corn flour
- ¼ cup fresh mint leaves
- 4 gloves garlic, crushed and chopped
- 1 inch ginger, chopped
- 3 green chilies, chopped
- 2 medium-sized potatoes, boiled and mashed
- 1 cup mixed vegetables, chopped
- Oil for brushing
- 12 pcs. bamboo skewers
- 1 tbsp. chaat masala
- Salt to taste

Instructions:
1) Placed the mixed vegetables, garlic, ginger, green chilies, and mint leaves in a food processor. Pulse until minced.
2) In a large mixing bowl, add the mixed vegetable mixture, mashed potatoes, garam masala powder, and corn flour. Season with salt to taste then mix well. This will be the kebab mixture.
3) Wet your palms and form balls around the bamboo skewer. Make sure that the kebab mixture adheres properly on the skewers so that they do not fall apart. Let it rest inside the fridge.
4) Meanwhile, preheat the air fryer to 392° Fahrenheit (200° Celsius) for 5 minutes.
5) Brush the kebab lightly with oil and fry at 356° Fahrenheit (180° Celsius) for 10 minutes or until brown.

13. Vegan Sabudana Vada

Serving Size: 2

Calories: 112 per serving

Ingredients:
- Salt to taste
- 2 tbsp. coriander leaves, chopped
- ½ tbsp. lemon juice
- 2 green chilies, chopped
- 1 tsp. grated ginger
- ¼ cup amaranth (rajgira) flour
- 1 cup potatoes, boiled and mashed
- ½ cup sago (sabudana) or tapioca

Instructions:
1) Wash the tapioca and drain. Let it rest for two hours while constantly sprinkling water to prevent it from drying.
2) Mix the tapioca with the other ingredients and knead to create a soft dough.
3) Divide the mixture into 12 portions and shape them into flat, round biscuits. Brush with oil and set aside.
4) Preheat the air fryer for 5 minutes at 392° Fahrenheit (200° Celsius).
5) Air fry the biscuits for 10 minutes until golden brown.

14. Hara Bhara Kabab

Serving Size: 1 to 2

Calories: 350 per serving

Ingredients:
- Oil for brushing
- Salt to taste
- 2 ½ tbsp. gram flour, roasted
- 1 tsp. ginger-green chili paste
- 1 tsp. dry mango powder
- 1 tsp. chaat masala powder
- ¾ cup peas
- 2 medium-sized potatoes, steamed and mashed
- 2 cups chopped spinach, blanched and drained

Instructions:
1) Preheat the oven to 392° Fahrenheit (200° Celsius) for 5 minutes.
2) In a mixing bowl, mix all ingredients together.
3) Divide the mixture and shape around bamboo skewers.
4) Brush lightly with oil and air fry for 10 minutes or until golden brown.

15. Curried Corn Balls

Serving Size: 10 medium-sized balls

Calories: 70 per ball

Ingredients:
- Salt and pepper to taste
- Oil for brushing
- Corn flour for binding
- 1 cup fresh corn, grated
- ½ cup black beans, chopped
- ½ cup carrots, chopped
- ¼ cup peas
- 2 medium-sized potatoes, boiled and mashed
- 2 tbsp. curry spice

Instructions:
1) In a mixing bowl, mix all ingredients except for the oil. Mix well to incorporate.
2) Shape the mixture into balls and lightly brush with oil.
3) Preheat the air fryer for 5 minutes at 356° Fahrenheit (180° Celsius).
4) Cook for 10 minutes or until golden brown.

16. Aalu Samosa

Serving Size: 10 small samosas

Calories: 138 per samosa

Ingredients:
- Water as needed
- Salt to taste
- Oil for brushing
- 1 tsp. anise seed powder
- ½ tsp. chana masala
- ½ tsp. turmeric powder
- 1 tsp. cumin seeds
- 3 tbsp. olive oil
- 2 tsp. coriander leaves, chopped
- 1 tsp. green chili, chopped
- ¼ cup peas
- 2 medium-sized potatoes, boiled and peeled
- 1 ½ cup white flour

Instructions:
1) In a bowl, mix together flour and olive oil. Add the water, anise, and salt. Knead to form a smooth dough. Let the dough rest for 30 minutes.
2) In a skillet, heat oil and add cumin seeds until it crackles. Add the turmeric powder, peas, green chili, and chana masala. Season with salt. Add the chopped potatoes and coriander leaves. Set aside.
3) Divide the dough into equal portions then roll out to flatten. Cut out a cone shape from the dough and fill it with the potato mixture.
4) Seal the dough by brushing the edges with water.
5) Brush the dough with oil, then air fry for 18 minutes in a 356º Fahrenheit (180º Celsius) preheated air fryer or until golden brown.

17. Chakli

Serving Size: 2

Calories: 475 per serving

Ingredients:
- Chakli press or any pastry mold
- Water as needed
- Salt to taste
- Oil for brushing
- 1 tsp. cumin powder
- 1 tsp. coriander powder
- ½ tsp. turmeric powder
- ½ tsp. red chili powder
- ½ tsp. sesame seeds
- 1 tbsp. olive oil
- ½ cup flour
- ½ cup roasted besan
- 1 cup rice flour

Instructions:
1) In a mixing bowl, combine the rice flour, refined flour, besan, turmeric powder, red chili powder, coriander powder, sesame seeds, cumin powder, and olive oil. Mix well, then add salt.
2) Add water and knead until you form a soft dough.
3) Preheat the air fryer for 5 minutes at 356º Fahrenheit (180º Celsius).
4) Place the dough into the chakli press. If you don't have a chakli press, you can use any cookie mold or just flatten the dough and cut out desired shapes.
5) Brush the dough with oil lightly.
6) Air fry for 12 minutes until golden brown.

18. Chana Dal Vada (2)

Serving Size: 1 to 2

Calories: 41 per serving

Ingredients:
- Water as needed
- Salt to taste
- Oil for brushing
- ¾ tsp. red chili powder
- 1 tsp. ginger, finely chopped
- 1 pc. green chili, chopped
- 2 tsp. coriander leaves, chopped
- 1 small onion, chopped
- 1 ½ cups chana daal

Instructions:
1) Wash the daal then soak in water for at least 2 hours.
2) Drain the daal and transfer to a blender until a coarse paste is formed.
3) Remove the daal from the food processor and transfer into a bowl.
4) Mix the coriander leaves, onion, ginger, green chili, red chili, and salt.
5) Divide the mixture into equal portions and flatten into small patties.
6) Brush with oil and cook in a preheated air fryer at 356° Fahrenheit (180° Celsius) or until golden brown.

19. Shahi Tukda

Serving Size: 3

Calories: 270 per serving

Ingredients:
- 1 tsp. green cardamom powder
- ½ cup chopped nuts, any kind
- ¼ cup brown sugar
- 1 cup almond milk
- 3 slices white bread

Instructions:
1) Preheat the air fryer for 3 minutes at 392° Fahrenheit (200° Celsius).
2) Place the bread slices in the air fryer and cook for 5 minutes or until toasted well.
3) Meanwhile, mix together sugar, milk, and cardamom powder in a skillet heated over a medium flame. Let it boil for 5 minutes or until the mixture thickens.
4) Remove the bread from the air fryer and top with the thickened milk mixture.
5) Garnish with mixed nuts of your choice.

20. Matar Kachodi

Serving Size: 1 to 2

Calories: 350 per serving

Ingredients:
- Water as needed
- Salt to taste
- Oil for brushing
- A pinch of baking soda
- ½ tsp. amchur powder
- ½ tsp. garam masala powder
- ½ tsp. red chili pepper
- 1 tsp. coriander powder
- ½ tsp. cumin seeds, roasted
- 3 tbsp. olive oil
- 1 tsp. green chili, chopped
- 1 tsp. ginger, chopped
- ½ cup peas, boiled
- ½ cup refined flour

Instructions:
1) In a mixing bowl, mix together flour, baking soda, and salt. Sift the mixture to remove lumps. Add olive oil and knead to make dough. Add water as needed.
2) In a skillet, heat oil and add cumin seeds and let it crackle. Add in the ginger, coriander powder, peas, green chili, red chili, garam masala, amchur, and salt. Mix well and sauté for 3-5 minutes. Set aside the filling mixture.
3) Roll the dough into a thin sheet and cut 4-inch squares.
4) Place the filling mixture at the center of the dough and fold as you would a wonton. Seal the edges with water. Brush the dough with oil lightly.
5) Air fry in a 356° Fahrenheit (180° Celsius) pre-heated air fryer for 18 minutes or until golden brown.

21. Gujiya

Serving Size: 2

Calories: 800 per serving

Ingredients:
- Oil for brushing
- 1 tsp. green cardamom powder
- ¼ cup powdered sugar
- 3 tbsp. raisins
- 3 tbsp. cashew nuts, chopped
- 3 tbsp. olive oil
- 1 cup white flour
- 1 cup vegan cheese, grated

Instructions:
1) Preheat the air fryer at 356° Fahrenheit (180° Celsius) for 5 minutes.
2) In a mixing bowl, mix together flour and oil. Add water as needed and knead to form a dough. Set aside.
3) In another bowl, mix the cashew nuts, vegan cheese, cardamom, raisins, and sugar until well combined.
4) Divide the dough into equal parts and roll out sheets of the dough. Place in a gujiya mold and add the filling in the middle. Press the mold and seal the edges with water.
5) Brush the gujiyas with oil.
6) Cook the gujiyas for 12 minutes or until golden brown.

22. Vegan-Style Pancakes

Serving Size: 8 pancakes

Calories: 10 per pancake

Ingredients:

- Soy yogurt, optional
- Jam for topping, optional
- Fresh fruit for topping, optional
- Cooking spray
- ½ tsp. vanilla
- 1 tbsp. maple syrup, plus more for serving
- 1 ¼ cups unsweetened plain soy milk
- ½ tsp. salt
- 2 tsp. baking powder
- 1 ¼ cups whole wheat flour

Instructions:

1) In a medium bowl, whisk together salt, baking powder, and flour.
2) In same bowl, pour in vanilla, maple syrup, and soy milk. Whisk well.
3) Insert your air fryer's nonstick baking dish pan and heat for a minute or two at 300º F.
4) Spray with cooking spray, pour in around ¼-cup of the batter, and cook for 2-3 minutes or until numerous bubbles form.
5) Flip pancake and cook the other side for a minute.
6) Repeat steps 4 and 5 until all the batter is used up.
7) Serve pancake with maple syrup on top. If desired, you can also add fresh fruit, jam, and soy yogurt as toppings to your pancake.

23. Baadal Jaam

Serving Size: 2

Calories: 118 per serving

Ingredients:
- Salt to taste
- Oil for brushing
- Coriander leaves for garnish
- 1 tsp. red chili powder
- 2 tsp. chaat masala
- 1 tsp. ginger garlic paste
- 1 lemon, juice-squeezed
- 2 big tomatoes, chopped
- 1 medium onion, chopped
- 1 medium round Brinjal
- ½ cup tofu curd

Instructions:
1) Cut the brinjal into ½ thick round sheets.
2) Preheat the air fryer at 392° Fahrenheit (200° Celsius) for 5 minutes. Air fry the brinjal for 8 minutes or until it is cooked through.
3) In a skillet, heat 2 tsp. oil and sauté the onions until golden brown. Add the tomatoes and ginger-garlic paste and cook for 3 more minutes.
4) Add the beaten tofu curd and cook. Add salt to taste as well as the red chili powder.
5) Assemble the brinjal by sprinkling lemon juice and chaat masala on top.
6) Spread the tomato and onion mixture and garnish with coriander leaves.

Mediterranean Recipes

24. Asparagus-Filled Phyllo Pastry

Serving Size: 2 to 4

Calories: 200 per serving

Ingredients:
- Salt and pepper to taste
- 2 tsp. whole mustard seed
- 1 tsp. capers, minced
- 1 tbsp. horseradish, grated
- ½ cup vegan mayonnaise
- ½ cup vegan parmesan cheese, grated
- 1 bunch green asparagus, trimmed
- 1 stick unsalted vegan butter, melted
- 1 package phyllo dough, defrosted

Instructions:
1) In a bowl, mix together vegan mayonnaise, capers, horseradish, and mustard. Add salt and pepper to taste. Set aside.
2) In a large pot, boil water and add salt. Blanch the trimmed asparagus for 2 minutes then drain and put in an ice water bath to prevent the asparagus from over cooking. Pat the asparagus dry using paper towels.
3) Place a phyllo sheet on top of a clean and damp kitchen towel to keep it from drying out. Brush with melted vegan butter or olive oil, then sprinkle vegan cheese and pepper. Repeat the process until you create 3 layers of phyllo sheets.
4) Divide the phyllo sheets into 5 equal strips so that you have 20 rectangles.
5) Place a stalk of asparagus on the bottom edge of the rectangle, then slowly roll. Brush the outside layer with vegan butter.
6) Place inside the preheated air fryer at 356° Fahrenheit (180° Celsius) and cook for 15 minutes.
7) Serve with the vegan mayonnaise sauce.

25. Spanakopita Bites

Serving Size: 2

Calories: 237 per serving

Ingredients:

- 2 tbsp. vegetable oil
- 8 tbsp. vegan butter, melted
- 1 pound phyllo dough, thawed
- Salt and pepper to taste
- ¼ cup silken tofu, blended until smooth
- 1 cup vegan cream cheese
- 6 ounces of vegan cheese, crumbled
- 10-ounces spinach, chopped
- 3 green onions, chopped
- 1 small onion, chopped
- 1 tablespoon vegetable oil

Instructions:

1) Preheat the air fryer to 375° Fahrenheit (190° Celsius).
2) In a skillet, heat 1 tablespoon oil over medium heat and sauté green and white onion until caramelized. Set aside.
3) In another bowl, mix together the vegan cheese, spinach, tofu, and the cooked onions. Season with salt and pepper. Set aside inside the refrigerator.
4) Combine the butter and remaining oil.
5) Remove the phyllo dough from the package and stack each sheet on one another. Cut the phyllo dough into two-inch squares.
6) Brush a mini muffin pan with vegan butter and place two squares of the phyllo dough on it. Push the dough down to create a crust. Brush the top with melted butter. Repeat the process until you create three layers of phyllo dough.
7) Place a spoonful of the filling into the cups and cook in the air fryer for 20 minutes or until golden brown.

26. Mediterranean Vegetables

Serving Size: 4

Calories: 100 per serving

Ingredients:
- Salt and pepper to taste
- 1 tbsp. olive oil
- 2 tsp. garlic puree
- 1 tsp. mustard
- 2 tbsp. agave syrup
- 1 tsp. mixed herbs of your choice
- 1 medium carrots, sliced
- 1 large parsnip, sliced
- 1 green pepper, sliced
- 1 large zucchini, sliced
- 1 cup cherry tomatoes, sliced

Instructions:
1) Place all sliced vegetables in a bowl.
2) Add in the rest of the ingredients and toss to coat the vegetable slices evenly.
3) Transfer the vegetables to the air fryer basket.
4) Cook in a preheated air fryer at 392° Fahrenheit (200° Celsius) for 5 minutes.
5) Transfer the cooked vegetables onto a baking tray and season with salt and pepper to adjust the taste.

27. Mediterranean Eggplant Chips

Serving Size: 15 chips

Calories: 13 per chip

Ingredients:
- 1 tbsp. extra virgin olive oil
- ¼ tsp. rosemary
- ½ tsp. salt
- ½ tsp. pepper, crushed
- ½ tsp. oregano
- ½ tsp. parsley, chopped
- ½ tsp. basil, chopped
- ½ of a large eggplant, sliced thinly

Instructions:
1) Preheat the air fryer to 392° Fahrenheit (200° Celsius) for 5 minutes.
2) Mix all the dry spices in a small mixing bowl. Add the extra virgin olive oil.
3) Pour the marinade over the eggplant slices and toss to coat everything.
4) Place the eggplant slices at the bottom of the air fryer basket and cook for 15 to 20 minutes.
5) Once the timer is off, let the eggplant chips rest inside the fryer until cool.

28. Mini Stuffed Grape Leaves Casserole

Serving Size: 3 to 4 mini casseroles

Calories: 100 per casserole

Ingredients:
- 1 lemon, sliced for garnish
- ¼ cup lemon juice
- 1 cup raisins or dried currants
- 1 cup fresh mint, chopped
- 1 cup parsley, chopped
- 1 cup hulled pistachios, chopped
- 2 cups tomato juice or vegetable juice
- 1 cup brown rice
- 1 large onion, diced
- 2 tbsp. olive oil
- 30 fresh grape leaves

Instructions:
1) Blanch the grape leaves in a boiling pot of water for 2 minutes. Drain, then set aside.
2) In a skillet, heat oil over medium heat and sauté onions for 10 minutes or until caramelized. Add uncooked brown rice and 2 ½ cups water and bring to a boil. Cover then reduce the heat to medium-low. Cook for 30 minutes until the liquid is absorbed by the rice.
3) Remove from heat and add in tomato juice, parsley, pistachios, mint, lemon juice, and raisins. Season with salt and pepper to taste.
4) Preheat the air fryer to 392° Fahrenheit (200° Celsius) for 5 minutes.
5) In a small ramekin, brush with olive oil. Line the bottom with grape leaves. Allow the leaves to hang over the sides of the ramekin. Spread the rice mixture. Top rice with more grape leaves. Brush with olive oil and air fry for 20 to 25 minutes or until the grape leaves wilt and the rice becomes dry.

29. Air-Fried Mediterranean Yellow Squash, Zucchini and Carrots

Serving Size: 2 to 3

Calories: 80 per serving

Ingredients:
- 1 tbsp. tarragon leaves, chopped
- ½ tsp. ground white pepper
- 1 tsp. salt
- 1 lb. yellow squash, cut into ¾ inch slices
- 1 lb. zucchini, cut into ¾ inch slices
- 2 tsp. olive oil
- ½ lb. carrots, peeled and cut into ¾ inch slices

Instructions:
1) In a bowl, combine the carrot with 2 tsp. of olive oil and toss. Place the carrots in a preheated air fryer at 400° Fahrenheit (204° Celsius) for 5 minutes.
2) While the carrots are cooking, place the yellow squash and zucchini in another bowl. Drizzle with the remaining olive oil and season with salt and pepper to taste. Toss to coat the vegetables. Once the carrots are done, remove them from the air fryer basket and put in the squash vegetables. Set the timer for 30 minutes.
3) Once the vegetables are done, toss all vegetables with tarragon.

30. Pesto-Potato Tofu Frittata Cups

Serving Size: 2 to 3

Calories: 420 per serving

Ingredients:
- ¼ cup nutritional yeast
- 1 block soft tofu
- 2 tbsp. all-purpose flour
- 2 tbsp. Dijon mustard
- 2 cloves garlic, peeled and crushed
- 2 cups leafy greens (basil leaves, parsley, arugula)
- 1 small red bell pepper, diced
- 1 small onion, diced
- 3 tbsp. olive oil, divided
- 1 large potato, sliced

Instructions:
1) In a skillet over medium heat, put 1 tablespoon olive oil and sauté the onions, bell pepper, and potatoes. Cook for 15 minutes until the vegetables turn slightly brown. Set aside to cool.
2) In a food processor, place the garlic and leafy greens, then pulse. Add the flour and mustard seed, then pulse until combined. Add the nutritional yeast and tofu and pulse until smooth.
3) Brush ramekins with oil. Place the potato mixture on the bottom layer and pour the tofu mixture.
4) Cook in an air fryer preheated at 392° Fahrenheit (200° Celsius) for 20 minutes or until a toothpick inserted in the middle comes out clean.

31. Crispy Brussel Sprouts with Garlic

Serving Size: 1

Calories: 249 per serving

Ingredients:
- Salt and pepper to taste
- 2 tbsp. rock salt
- 2 tbsp. olive oil
- 2 garlic cloves, sliced
- 10 small Brussels sprouts, cleaned and rinsed

Instructions:
1) Bring a pot of water to a boil, then add salt. Blanch the Brussels sprouts for 4 minutes, then shock in cold water to stop the cooking process.
2) Cut the Brussels sprouts lengthwise.
3) In a mixing bowl, combine all the ingredients and toss to coat the Brussels sprouts lightly.
4) Cook for 15 minutes in a preheated air fryer at 392° Fahrenheit (200° Celsius).

32. Vegan Mushroom Meatballs

Serving Size: 20 meatballs

Calories: 70 per meatball

Ingredients:
- Parsley for garnish
- 1 24-oz. can marinara sauce
- 3 tbsp. olive oil
- ¼ tsp. pepper
- ¼ tsp. salt
- ½ tsp. dried thyme
- ½ tsp. dried oregano
- ½ block firm tofu, crumbled
- 4 cloves garlic, minced
- ½ cup chopped parsley
- 1 cup breadcrumbs
- 1 cup quick oats
- 20 oz. mushrooms, chopped
- 1 medium onion, chopped

Instructions:
1) In a skillet, heat the olive oil on medium-low heat and sauté the onions for 7 minutes.
2) Add the mushrooms and cook for another 15 minutes or until the moisture evaporates and the mushrooms turn brown. Add the garlic and transfer the mixture to a bowl. Set aside.
3) Add the remaining ingredients (except the marinara sauce) to another bowl. Mix until well combined then refrigerate for 2 hours.
4) Form small balls from the mushroom mixture.
5) Preheat the air fryer to 392° Fahrenheit (200° Celsius) for 5 minutes. Cook the mushroom balls for 15 minutes or until golden brown.
6) Meanwhile, heat up the marinara sauce. Pour marinara sauce over cooked mushroom balls. Garnish with parsley.

33. Mediterranean Spiced Carrots

Serving Size: 3 to 4

Calories: 100 per serving

Ingredients:
- 1 tsp. salt
- ½ tsp. red pepper flakes
- 2 tsp. dried oregano
- 2 tsp. dried basil
- 1 tsp. dried rosemary
- 3 tsp. dried parsley
- 2 tbsp. olive oil
- 2 lbs. carrots, peeled and cut into large strips

Instructions:
1) Preheat the air fryer to 392° Fahrenheit (200° Celsius) for 5 minutes.
2) In a bowl, mix together the first five ingredients.
3) Add the olive oil and carrots. Toss to coat the carrots with the seasoning.
4) Air fry for 20 minutes until golden brown and tender.

34. Greek Spinach "Meatloaf" Cups

Serving Size: 5 to 6

Calories: 147 per serving

Ingredients:
- ¼ cup pine nuts
- ¼ cup ketchup
- 1 tsp. Worcestershire sauce
- ¼ tsp. salt
- ¼ tsp. black pepper
- ½ tsp. dried thyme
- ½ tsp. dried parsley
- ½ tsp. dried oregano
- 1 tbsp. flaxseed meal mixed with 3 tbsp. water
- ⅓ cup seasoned bread crumbs
- 3 tbsp. flour
- ¼ cup chopped yellow onions
- ⅓ cup diced red peppers, roasted
- ½ cup tofu, crumbled
- 4 cups baby spinach
- 2 cloves minced garlic
- 1 tsp. olive oil

Instructions:
1) Preheat the air fryer to 400° Fahrenheit (204° Celsius).
2) Grease the ramekins with olive oil, then set aside.
3) In a skillet, heat oil over medium-low heat and sauté garlic with the baby spinach. Cook until the spinach wilts. Set aside.
4) In a mixing bowl, add all ingredients and combine with your hands.
5) Dump the mixture into greased ramekins and brush top with ketchup.
6) Air fry for 25 minutes until a toothpick inserted comes out clean.
7) Cook until all batches are finished.

35. Roasted Beets with Lemon Vinaigrette

Serving Size: 3

Calories: 69 per serving

Ingredients:

- ¼ cup chopped fresh Italian parsley
- ¼ tsp. black pepper, ground
- ¼ tsp. salt
- 1 tsp. Dijon mustard
- 1 clove garlic, minced
- 2 tsp. fresh lemon juice
- 2 tbsp. extra virgin olive oil
- 6 beets, trimmed and sliced

Instructions:

1) Preheat the air fryer to 400° Fahrenheit (204° Celsius).
2) Air fry the beets for 25 minutes until tender.
3) Meanwhile, mix the rest of the ingredients.
4) Drizzle over the beets and garnish with Italian parsley.

36. Vegan Calzone

Serving Size: 2

Calories: 300 per serving

Ingredients:

For the dough
- 1 tsp. caster sugar
- 2 tsp. dried active yeast
- 1 tsp. salt
- 12 oz. white bread flour

For the tomato sauce
- 1 tbsp. tomato puree
- 1 tsp. oregano
- 1 tsp. sugar
- 1 cup chopped tomatoes
- 2 cloves garlic, peeled and crushed
- 1 tbsp. olive oil

For the filling
- 4 oz. vegan cashew mozzarella, crumbled
- 2 tbsp. olive oil
- 1 small eggplant, cut into small chunks
- 1 zucchini, cut into small chunks
- 1 red, orange, and yellow pepper, cut into small chunks

Instructions:
1) Prepare the dough by mixing all ingredients together. Let the dough rise for 30 minutes to an hour before rolling it into a round pizza dough. Let it rest.
2) Prepare the tomato sauce by heating the olive oil in a skillet over medium flame and sautéing the tomatoes and garlic. Add the rest of the ingredients and let the sauce simmer for 5 minutes. Set aside.
3) Prepare the toppings by lightly coating the vegetables with oil.
4) Preheat the air fryer to 400° Fahrenheit (204° Celsius) for 5 minutes.
5) Add the vegetables and air fry for 10 minutes.
6) Assemble the calzone by putting tomato sauce on the dough and the vegetable filling.
7) Seal the dough tightly and put inside the air fryer. Cook for 20 minutes or until the dough becomes golden brown.

37. Best Herb Roast Potatoes

Serving Size: 4

Calories: 138.50 per serving

Ingredients:

For the herbed oil
- Salt and pepper to taste
- 3 tbsp. mixed fresh herbs like thyme, parsley, oregano, and basil
- ¼ cup olive oil

For the potatoes
- 1 tbsp. olive oil
- ¼ tsp. pepper
- ¼ tsp. salt
- 2 lbs. mini potatoes

Instructions:

1) Preheat the air fryer to 400° Fahrenheit (204° Celsius) for 5 minutes.
2) Place the potatoes on a counter and make thin slices on the potatoes. Make sure that the slices do not go all the way through so the potatoes are still intact.
3) Toss the tomatoes with a little bit of salt and pepper. Add the olive oil.
4) Roast in the air fryer for 25 minutes until the potatoes are crispy on the outside and tender on the inside.
5) Prepare the herbed dressing by mixing all ingredient together. Pour the dressing over the potatoes once cooked.

38. Artichoke Basil Toasts

Serving Size: 10 toasts

Calories: 19 per toast

Ingredients:

- 10 small pieces of whole wheat bread
- 2 cups fresh baby spinach
- 1 cup jarred artichoke hearts, drained
- Salt and pepper to taste
- A drizzle of olive oil
- Juice of one lemon
- A handful of fresh basil
- 1 14 oz. can of chickpeas
- 1 clove garlic

Instructions:

1) Toast the bread in the air fryer at 400° Fahrenheit (204° Celsius) for 5 minutes. Set aside.
2) In a food processor, pulse the chickpeas and garlic. Add the basil and continue pulsing until crumbly.
3) Transfer the chickpea mixture into a bowl and add in chopped artichokes, lemon juice, and olive oil. Season with salt and pepper to taste.
4) Add the spinach greens.
5) Top the toasted bread with the chickpea mixture.

39. Turmeric Roasted Cauliflower Salad with Lemon Tahini Dressing

Serving Size: 4

Calories: 100 per serving

Ingredients:

Ingredients:

For toasted cauliflower
- 1 tsp. rapeseed oil
- A dash of coriander and garlic powder
- ½ tsp. turmeric powder
- Salt and pepper
- 1 head cauliflower, cut into florets

For tahini dressing
- ¼ cup pomegranate seeds
- ¼ cup pine nuts, roasted
- Fresh parsley for garnish
- ½ tsp. maple syrup
- Water as needed
- ¼ lemon, juiced
- Salt and pepper to taste
- 1 clove garlic, crushed
- 1 tsp. rapeseed oil
- 1 tbsp. tahini

Instructions:

1) Preheat the air fryer to 356° Fahrenheit (180° Celsius) for 5 minutes.
2) In a bowl, toss all the ingredients for the toasted cauliflower and roast in the air fryer for 25 minutes.
3) Make the dressing by combining all the ingredients together, except for the pomegranate, pine nuts, and fresh parsley.
4) Once the cauliflower is done, sprinkle with the pomegranate, pine nuts, and parsley. Drizzle with the tahini dressing.

40. Sautéed Carrots and Shallots with Thyme

Serving Size: 4

Calories: 150 per serving

Ingredients:
- Pepper to taste
- ½ tsp. salt
- 1 to 2 tbsp. fresh thyme, chopped
- 2 tbsp. salted vegan butter or olive oil
- 1 cup vegetable broth
- 4 to 5 shallots, chopped
- 12 medium carrots, peeled and sliced

Instructions:
1) In a skillet, heat the oil or vegan butter and sauté the shallots. Add the carrots and the broth.
2) Let it simmer for a few minutes until the sauce thickens a bit.
3) Remove the carrots from the sauce and transfer them to a mixing bowl. Add the rest of the ingredients.
4) Preheat the air fryer to 356° Fahrenheit (180° Celsius) for 5 minutes.
5) Air fry the carrots for 8 minutes or until the carrots are crisp tender and the sides are brown.
6) Serve the carrots with the thickened sauce.

41. Stuffed Mushrooms

Serving Size: 2

Calories: 271 per serving

Ingredients:

- ¼ cup grated vegan cheese
- ½ cup panko
- 1 tsp. Greek seasoning
- 2 cups fresh spinach, chopped
- 2 cloves garlic, minced
- 1 onion, chopped fine
- 1 red bell pepper, chopped fine
- 1 tbsp. olive oil
- 2 8-oz. cans whole mushrooms, stems removed and chopped for the filling

Instructions:

1) Heat oil in a skillet over medium flame and sauté the red pepper, garlic, onion, and mushroom stems. Add the Greek seasoning and continue to cook for 8 minutes. Add chopped spinach until wilted. Set aside to cool.
2) In a mixing bowl, mix the sautéed vegetables with the vegan cheese and panko.
3) Preheat the air fryer to 356° Fahrenheit (180° Celsius) for 5 minutes.
4) Place the mushrooms cap-side down and put filling in the hollowed-out part where the stems used to be.
5) Cook for 25 minutes in the air fryer until lightly browned.

Asian Recipes

42. Avocado Tempura

Serving Size: 4

Calories: 103 per serving

Ingredients:
- Aquafaba from one 15-oz. can of garbanzo beans (liquid of garbanzo beans)
- 1 large peeled avocado, pitted and sliced
- ½ tsp. salt
- ½ cup panko bread

Instructions:
1) In a bowl, toss the panko and salt. Set aside.
2) In another bowl, pour the garbanzo bean liquid. Set aside.
3) Dredge the avocado slices in the aquafaba before dipping in the panko mixture.
4) Arrange the avocado slices inside the fryer basket. Do not overlap them.
5) Air fry for 10 minutes at 390° Fahrenheit (about 200° Celsius). Shake the basket midway through the cooking process. There's no need to preheat the fryer.
6) Serve with your favorite dipping sauce.

43. Sesame Toast

Serving Size: 3 toasts

Calories: 117 per toast

Ingredients:
- Salt and pepper to taste
- Oil for brushing
- Sesame seeds for coating
- 2 tbsp. refined flour
- 2 tbsp. corn flour
- ¼ cup peas, boiled
- ¼ cup beans, chopped
- 1 potato, boiled and mashed
- 3 slices white bread

Instructions:
1) In a mixing bowl, mix together carrots, peas, beans, and mashed potatoes. Season with salt and pepper to taste.
2) Cut the bread slices into 4 parts and put the vegetable mixture on top.
3) In another bowl, combine the corn flour and refined flour. Add water to make a thick paste.
4) Coat the bread slices with the flour mixture and sprinkle with sesame seeds on top. Brush with oil on top.
5) Preheat the air fryer for five minutes at 392° Fahrenheit (200° Celsius) and cook for 5 minutes.

44. Coconut Tofu

Serving Size: 4

Calories: 183 per serving

Ingredients:
- Olive oil for brushing
- 1 ½ cups unsweetened coconut, shredded
- 1 block firm tofu, pressed then cut into one-inch fingers
- ¼ cup flax meal
- ¾ cup water

Instructions:
1) Preheat the air fryer to 392° Fahrenheit (200° Celsius) for 5 minutes.
2) In a bowl, mix together water and flax meal and set it aside for 5 minutes for the mixture to thicken.
3) In another bowl, pour the shredded coconut.
4) Coat the tofu slices in the flax mixture first before dipping in the shredded coconut.
5) Arrange in layers at the bottom of the air fryer basket. Brush with oil.
6) Air fry for 20 minutes. Make sure that you flip the tofu every 10 minutes.
7) Cook until golden brown.

45. Katsu Banh Mi

Serving Size: 4 banh mi

Calories: 287 per banh mi

Ingredients:

For aioli
- 2 tsp. coarse sugar
- 2 tbsp. vegan Worcestershire sauce
- 2 tbsp. ketchup
- ¼ cup vegan mayonnaise

For pickles
- 1 medium peeled cucumber, seeded and sliced
- ¼ cup rice vinegar
- ½ tsp. sea salt
- 1 tbsp. coarse sugar
- ¼ cup hot water

For tofu
- ½ tsp. dried sage
- ½ tsp. dried thyme
- ½ tsp. sea salt
- 1 tsp. dried parsley
- 3 tbsp. nutritional yeast
- 2 cups water
- 1 14-oz. package of firm tofu, pressed to remove moisture

For katsu
- 1 tsp. ginger, grated
- 1 tsp. garlic, minced
- ¼ cup all-purpose flour
- 6 tbsp. aquafaba or non-dairy milk
- 1 cup panko bread crumbs

For sandwich
- Cilantro for garnish
- Slices of jalapeno for garnish
- 4 banh mi rolls

Instructions:

1) For the aioli: combine all ingredients in a mixing bowl. Set aside.
2) For pickles: prepare a few days before by mixing all ingredients except the cucumber to make the brine. Place the cucumbers in the brine and let ferment for 3 days.

3) For the tofu: cut the tofu into ½-inch thick slices. In a pan, heat the remaining ingredients and bring to a boil. Add the tofu slices and let them simmer for 10 minutes. Marinade for 3 days in the fridge.
4) For the katsu: combine all ingredients together.
5) Dredge the marinated tofu into the katsu mixture. Brush with oil and cook in a preheated air fryer at 390° Fahrenheit (199° Celsius) for 15 minutes or until golden brown.
6) Assemble the sandwiches by toasting the bread. Place the tofu tonkatsu on top of the bread then spread the aioli mixture on top of the tofu. Add the cucumber pickles. Garnish with jalapeno and cilantro.

46. Air-Fried Tofu Scramble

Serving Size: 4

Calories: 139 per serving

Ingredients:

- 4 cups broccoli florets
- 1 tbsp. olive oil
- 2 ½ cups red potato, chopped into 1-inch cubes
- ½ cup onions, chopped
- ½ tsp. garlic powder
- ½ tsp. onion powder
- 1 tsp. turmeric
- 1 tbsp. soy sauce
- 1 block of tofu, chopped into 1-inch cubes

Instructions:

1) In a medium bowl, toss the tofu, olive oil, soy sauce, garlic powder, turmeric, onion powder, and chopped onions. Set aside.
2) In another bowl, combine the potatoes and olive oil and air fry at 400° Fahrenheit (204° Celsius) for 15 minutes. Shake the fryer basket halfway through the cooking time.
3) Add the marinated tofu and cook for 15 minutes at 370° Fahrenheit (188° Celsius).
4) Meanwhile, cook the broccoli with the remaining marinade on a skillet over medium heat. Set aside.
5) Serve the potatoes and tofu with the broccoli.

47. Crispy Trumpet Mushroom Tempura

Serving Size: 4

Calories: 111 per serving

Ingredients:
- Spiced coconut vinegar as dipping sauce
- Fresh parsley for garnish
- Lemon wedges for garnish
- A pinch of salt
- 1 cup non-dairy milk
- A pinch of chili pepper
- A dash of garlic powder
- ½ cup panko bread crumbs
- ½ cup flour
- 11-ounces trumpet mushroom
- Oil for brushing

Instructions:
1) Cut the mushroom into small trips.
2) In a mixing bowl, combine garlic powder, chili pepper, salt, bread crumbs, and flour. Set aside.
3) Dunk the mushroom in milk then coat with the flour mixture.
4) Place in the air fryer basket and brush with oil.
5) Air fry at 400° Fahrenheit (204° Celsius) for 15 minutes or until golden brown and crispy. Shake the fryer basket halfway through the cooking time.
6) Garnish with parsley and lemon wedges.
7) Dip in spiced coconut vinegar.

48. Spring Rolls

Serving Size: 10 to 15 spring rolls

Calories: 125 per spring roll

Ingredients:

- Salt to taste
- Oil for brushing
- 1 tsp. ginger, grated
- ½ cup cabbage, shredded
- ½ cup carrots, julienned
- 1 small onion, chopped finely
- 2 tbsp. soy sauce
- Seasoning to taste
- ½ block firm tofu, fried then chopped
- 1 tsp. corn flour
- 1 tsp. refined flour
- Spring roll sheets

Instructions:

1) In a bowl, mix the refined flour, corn flour, and soy sauce.
2) In a skillet, sauté the onions, cabbage, carrots, and ginger. Add the fried tofu then add the flour mixture to thicken. Add seasoning to taste. Let it simmer until the vegetable mixture dries.
3) Place the vegetable filling in the middle of the spring roll sheet, then roll. Seal the edges with water.
4) Brush lightly with oil and cook in the air fryer for 5 minutes at 356° Fahrenheit (180° Celsius) or until the spring rolls become golden brown and crispy.

49. Fried Garlic Mushroom

Serving Size: 2

Calories: 125 per serving

Ingredients:
- Oil for brushing
- Bread crumbs to coat
- 1 tbsp. flax seed mixed with 3 tbsp. water
- 1 tsp. coriander leaves, chopped
- 1 tsp. garlic, minced
- 1 tbsp. olive oil
- 1 can mushrooms
- Salt and pepper to taste
- toothpicks

Instructions:
1) In a bowl, add oil, garlic, coriander, and mushrooms. Season with salt and pepper to taste.
2) Using a toothpick, join two mushroom caps together.
3) Dip the mushrooms in the flaxseed mixture, then roll in bread crumbs. Brush surface with oil.
4) Preheat the air fryer to 392° Fahrenheit (200° Celsius) and cook for 10 minutes.

50. Fried Tofu with Sesame-Soy Dipping Sauce

Serving Size: 4

Calories: 163 per serving

Ingredients:

For the fried tofu
- ½ cup panko bread crumbs
- 1 tbsp. flax meal mixed with 3 tbsp. water
- ¼ tsp. ground white pepper
- ½ cup corn starch
- 1 block extra firm tofu, sliced and pressed

For the dipping sauce
- A dash of sesame seeds
- 1 spring onion, chopped
- 1 red chili pepper, minced
- 3 cloves garlic, chopped
- 2 tsp. sesame oil
- 1 tsp. sugar
- 1 tsp. rice wine vinegar
- ¼ cup soy sauce

Instructions:
1) In a bowl, mix the cornstarch and white pepper.
2) Put the panko bread crumbs in another bowl.
3) Coat the tofu slices with the cornstarch mixture followed by the flaxseed before dipping them into the panko crumbs.
4) Lightly brush the tofu with oil.
5) Air fry at 400° Fahrenheit (204° Celsius) for 15 minutes or until golden brown and crispy. Shake the fryer basket halfway through the cooking time.
6) Meanwhile, prepare the dipping sauce by mixing all the ingredients together.

51. Spicy Vegan Peanut Butter Tofu with Sriracha Sauce

Serving Size: 4

Calories: 130 per serving

Ingredients:

For tofu

- 3 tbsp. green onions, diagonally sliced
- 1 large ginger root, sliced
- 5 cloves of garlic, sliced
- 1 tbsp. peanut oil
- 16 oz. firm tofu, drained and sliced

For the sauce

- 1 tbsp. or more sriracha sauce
- 2 tbsp. vegetable stock
- 1 tbsp. agave nectar
- 2 tbsp. smooth natural peanut butter
- 3 tbsp. rice vinegar
- 3 tbsp. soy sauce

Instructions:

1) In a bowl, mix the rice vinegar, soy sauce, agave, peanut butter, stock, and sriracha sauce. Set aside.
2) Preheat the air fryer to 400° Fahrenheit (204° Celsius) for 5 minutes.
3) Cook the tofu in the air fryer for 25 minutes or until golden brown.
4) Heat a skillet over high heat and add peanut oil. Sauté ginger and garlic until fragrant. Add the air-fried tofu and cook for 3 minutes.
5) Add the sauce and simmer until it thickens.
6) Garnish with green onions.

52. General Tso's Baked Cauliflower

Serving Size: 4

Calories: 136 per serving

Ingredients:

For the cauliflower
- 4 green onions, sliced
- 1 tbsp. sesame seeds
- 1 tbsp. cornstarch
- 1 tsp. grapeseed oil
- 1 large cauliflower, cut into florets

For the sauce
- ½ tsp. cornstarch
- ½ tsp. chili flakes
- 1 tsp. sesame oil
- 2 tbsp. rice vinegar
- 2 tbsp. soy sauce
- 2 tbsp. agave or maple syrup
- ¼ cup hoisin sauce
- 3 cloves garlic, minced
- 1 tbsp. ginger, minced
- 1 tsp. grapeseed oil

Instructions:
1) Preheat the air fryer to 420° Fahrenheit (216° Celsius).
2) In a large bowl, place the cauliflower florets and toss with cornstarch and grapeseed oil.
3) Cook the cauliflower in an air fryer for 30 minutes, turning it over halfway through to cook evenly.
4) Meanwhile, sauté over medium heat ginger and garlic and cook for 2 minutes. Add the remaining ingredients and bring to a boil. Lower the heat until the sauce thickens.
5) Once the cauliflower is cooked, remove from the air fryer and pour sauce over the cauliflower. Sprinkle with sesame seeds and green onions.
6) Serve with rice.

53. Stick Sesame Cauliflower

Serving Size: 8

Calories: 243 per serving

Ingredients:
- Cooked rice
- Toasted sesame seeds for garnish
- 2 scallions, chopped
- ¼ cup cold water
- 1 tbsp. corn starch
- 1 tsp. sriracha
- 2 garlic cloves, minced
- 2 tsp. ginger, grated
- 2 tsp. sesame oil
- ¼ cup rice vinegar
- ½ cup maple syrup
- ½ cup soy sauce
- 1 large cauliflower, cut into florets
- ½ tsp. baking powder
- ½ tsp. salt
- 1 cup whole wheat flour
- 1 ¼ cups almond milk
- 1 tbsp. vegetable oil

Instructions:
1) Preheat the air fryer to 420° Fahrenheit (216° Celsius) for 5 minutes.
2) In bowl, combine almond milk, salt, flour, and baking powder.
3) Dip the cauliflower florets in the batter and shake off the excess batter.
4) Cook in the air fryer for 15 to 20 minutes.
5) Meanwhile, mix the soy sauce, rice vinegar, maple syrup, sesame oil, garlic, ginger, and sriracha in a small saucepan. Allow to simmer for 10 minutes. Add the cornstarch and let it thicken.
6) Remove the cauliflower from the air fryer and coat with the sauce. Add sesame seeds.
7) Serve with rice.

54. Air Fried Green Beans with Garlic Sauce

Serving Size: 2

Calories: 62 per serving

Ingredients:
- ½ tsp. corn starch
- ½ lb. green beans, trimmed at the end
- 2 cloves of garlic, chopped
- ½ tsp. sesame oil
- ¼ cup vegetable broth
- 1 tbsp. soy sauce

Instructions:
1) In a bowl, mix the soy sauce, broth, and sesame oil. Set aside.
2) Wash the beans and marinate in the soy sauce mixture for at least 24 hours.
3) Preheat the air fryer to 392° Fahrenheit (200° Celsius) for 5 minutes.
4) Sprinkle the beans with garlic and cook in the air fryer for 15 minutes.

55. Fried Ganmodoki

Serving Size: 15 fritters

Calories: 109 per fritter

Instructions:
- Salt and pepper to taste
- 50 grams of Hijiki seaweed, rehydrated
- 2 stalks green onion, sliced
- ¼ of one large carrot, julienned
- 250 grams okara (tofu skin)
- 2 blocks firm tofu

Ingredients:
1) Mix okara and tofu in a bowl.
2) Add the carrots, hijiki, and green onions. Season with salt and pepper to taste.
3) Make patties from the mixture and cook in an air fryer preheated to 356° Fahrenheit (180° Celsius) for 15 minutes or until golden brown.

56. Vegan Katsu Curry

Serving Size: 6

Calories: 178 per serving

Ingredients:

For the eggplant katsu
- 2 tbsp. sesame seeds
- 100 grams of panko bread crumbs
- 1 cup aquafaba
- Salt and pepper to taste
- ½ cup all-purpose flour
- 1 sweet potato, peeled
- 1 large eggplant, sliced

For the curry sauce
- 2 tsp. mirin
- 2 tsp. rice wine
- 4 tsp. soy sauce
- 1 tsp. garam masala
- 4 tsp. curry powder
- 1 tsp. white miso paste
- ½ granny smith apple, peeled and diced
- 2 medium carrots, peeled and sliced
- 3 tsp. ginger, grated
- 5 cloves garlic, diced
- 1 large onion, diced
- 2 tbsp. oil

Instructions:

1) Prepare the sauce by heating up the 2 tablespoons of oil in a pan. Sauté the onions until transparent, then add the garlic and continue cooking for a minute before mixing the ginger. Add the apples and carrots. Season with curry powder and garam masala. Continue to cook for 2 minutes.
2) In a small bowl, dissolve miso paste in 1 cup water. Add to the pan. Let it simmer on low heat for 15 minutes until the vegetables are soft.
3) Transfer the vegetable mixture to a blender and process until smooth. Season with soy sauce, mirin, and rice vinegar. Add water if the sauce is too thick.
4) Set the sauce aside, then prepare the eggplant katsu.
5) Prepare 4 plates. Pour ½ cup of flour (seasoned with salt and pepper) onto the first plate. Pour the aquafaba onto the second plate. The third plate should contain bread crumbs

with sesame seeds. Lastly, the fourth plate should only have a double layer of paper towels where the coated eggplants will rest before air frying.
6) Dredge the eggplant with the flour, followed by the aquafaba, then the panko. Let rest on the fourth plate for at least 1 hour in the fridge.
7) Preheat the air fryer to 392º Fahrenheit (200º Celsius) for 5 minutes.
8) Set the eggplants in the fryer basket and cook for 20 minutes. Flipping the eggplants halfway through the cooking time.

57. Crispy Kung Pao Cauliflower

Serving Size: 2

Calories: 168 per serving

Ingredients:

For the crispy cauliflower
- 1 medium-sized head cauliflower, cut into florets
- 1 tsp. oil
- ¼ tsp. roasted sesame oil
- ¼ tsp. salt
- 2 tsp. soy sauce
- ½ tsp. cayenne pepper
- ¼ cup + more water
- ¼ cup + more bread crumbs
- ¼ cup + more corn starch

For the kung pao sauce
- 2 tbsp. scallions, chopped
- 1 inch ginger, minced
- 5 cloves garlic, minced
- 3 tbsp. chopped peanuts
- ½ tsp. crushed Sichuan peppercorns
- 10 dried red chilies
- 1 tsp. oil
- 1 tsp. corn starch
- ¼ cup + more water
- 1 tbsp. sugar
- 1 tsp. Chinese rice wine
- 1 ½ tbsp. rice vinegar
- 2 ½ tbsp. soy sauce

Instructions:
1) Preheat the air fryer to 400° Fahrenheit (204° Celsius).
2) In a bowl, mix the bread crumbs and the rest of the ingredients for the crispy cauliflower to make a batter. Let the batter rest and adjust the water if it is too thick.
3) Dip the cauliflower in the batter and tap to remove the excess batter.
4) Cook in the air fryer for 30 minutes or until the cauliflower florets are cooked through.
5) Meanwhile, make the sauce by sautéing the peppercorns and chilies in an oiled skillet heated over a medium flame. Make sure that the red chilies do not turn too brown. Add the nuts, garlic, and ginger and reduce the heat to medium-low. Continue to cook for 5 minutes, stirring constantly.

6) Add the scallions and green peppers. Mix the remaining kung pao sauce ingredients and continue to cook. Adjust the seasoning to your liking.
7) Once the cauliflowers are cooked, place them in a bowl and drizzle with the sauce.

58. Eggplant with Garlic Sauce

Serving Size: 2

Calories: 61 per serving

Ingredients:
- 3 cloves garlic, chopped
- 1 tsp. ginger, grated
- 2 ½ tbsp. peanut oil
- 2 tsp. sugar
- ½ tsp. soy sauce
- 1 tsp. corn starch
- ¼ tsp. salt
- 2 Chinese eggplants, chopped

Instructions:
1) Place the eggplants in a bowl and add water with a little salt. Let it sit in the brine for 15 minutes, then drain and pat dry.
2) Spread the eggplants onto a paper towel and sprinkle with cornstarch. Let rest for 60 minutes.
3) In another bowl, combine the soy sauce, sugar, and cornstarch and mix well.
4) Go back to the eggplant and brush oil lightly.
5) Preheat the air fryer to 400° Fahrenheit (204° Celsius) for 5 minutes.
6) Cook the eggplants for 20 minutes or until the sides have been browned. Set aside once cooked.
7) In a skillet, heat the sauce mixture until it thickens. Add the remaining ingredients.
8) Pour over the air-fried eggplant.
9) Serve with water.

59. Asian-Style Tofu Burgers

Serving Size: 4 patties

Calories: 260 per patty

Ingredients:

For the tofu burgers
- 1 tbsp. olive oil
- ½ tsp. ground ginger
- ½ tsp. coriander
- 1 tsp. onion powder
- 1 tsp. garlic powder
- 4 tsp. soy sauce
- 1 tsp. minced ginger
- 2 tbsp. corn flour
- 1 cup bread crumbs
- 14 oz. extra firm tofu, drained and crumbled

For the BBQ sauce
- 1 tbsp. soy sauce
- 1 tsp. ground ginger powder
- 2 tsp. sriracha sauce
- ½ cup vegan French dressing (optional)
- ½ cup ketchup

Instructions:

1) In a bowl, mix all the ingredients for making tofu burgers. Mix well.
2) Form patties from the mixture and brush with oil.
3) Preheat the air fryer at 400° Fahrenheit (204° Celsius) for 5 minutes.
4) Cook the patties for 20 to 25 minutes or until golden brown.
5) Meanwhile, make the barbecue sauce by mixing all of the ingredients together.
6) Once the burgers are cooked, drizzle with the sauce and add additional toppings like sweet potato fries, tomatoes, and arugula.
7) Serve on a bun.

60. Air-Fried Sichuan Potstickers (Gyoza)

Serving Size: 24 dumplings

Calories: 104 per dumpling

Ingredients:

For the potstickers
- Oil for brushing
- 24 gyoza wrappers
- ½ tsp. ginger, grated
- ¼ tsp. garlic powder
- 1 tsp. dried scallions
- 1 tsp. Sichuan peppercorns
- 1 tsp. dried onion flakes
- 1 tbsp. hoisin sauce
- 4 cups Napa cabbage, sliced
- 8 oz. baby bella mushrooms, minced
- 2 tsp. sesame oil

For the dipping sauce
- ¼ tsp. dried scallions
- ¼ tsp. red pepper flakes
- 1 tbsp. rice wine vinegar
- 2 tbsp. soy sauce

Instructions:

1) In a skillet, heat the sesame oil over medium heat and sauté the mushrooms until golden brown. Add the cabbages until wilted. Add in the onion flakes, hoisin sauce, peppers, garlic powder, ginger, and scallions. Cook for another 3 minutes, then set aside to cool.
2) While the filling is cooling, prepare the sauce by combining all the ingredients in a small bowl.
3) Prepare the gyoza wrappers and add a teaspoon of the cooled filling at the center of each wrapper. Dip a finger in water and run it along the edges of the gyoza. Pinch the sides until you seal the dumpling.
4) Preheat the air fryer at 400° Fahrenheit (204° Celsius) for 5 minutes.
5) Place the dumplings on a small baking pan brushed with a little bit of oil.
6) Cook in the air fryer for 10 to 15 minutes.
7) Serve with the prepared dipping sauce.

American Recipes

61. Roasted Sweet Potatoes with Agave and Cinnamon

Serving Size: 4

Calories: 163 per serving

Ingredients:
- Salt and pepper to taste
- 2 tsp. ground cinnamon
- ¼ cup agave or maple syrup
- ¼ cup extra virgin olive oil
- 4 sweet potatoes, peeled and cut into 1-inch cubes

Instructions:
1) Preheat the air fryer to 392° Fahrenheit (200° Celsius).
2) In a mixing bowl, combine all ingredients and toss to coat all sweet potato cubes evenly.
3) Air fry the sweet potatoes for 30 minutes or until tender.
4) Drizzle with extra virgin olive oil if preferred.

62. Apple Dumplings

Serving Size: 2

Calories: 102 per serving

Ingredients:
- 2 tbsp. vegan butter, melted
- 2 sheets of puff pastry
- 1 tbsp. brown sugar
- 2 tbsp. raisins
- 1 small apple, cored and sliced

Instructions:
1) Preheat the air fryer to 392° Fahrenheit (200° Celsius).
2) In a bowl, mix the raisins and sugar. Set aside.
3) Place slices of apple on one puff pastry sheet, then fill with the raisins.
4) Using another pastry sheet, cover the top of the apple slices, then seal the edges.
5) Place the apple dumpling on aluminum foil and brush the dough with melted vegan butter.
6) Cook in the air fryer for 25 minutes or until the puff pastry dough turns brown.

63. Air-Fried Buffalo Cauliflower

Serving Size: 4

Calories: 132 per serving

Ingredients:
- Vegan mayonnaise for dipping
- ¼ cup vegan buffalo sauce
- ¼ cup melted vegan butter
- 1 cup panko bread crumbs
- 1 tsp. salt
- 4 cups cauliflower florets

Instructions:
1) In a mixing bowl, mix together panko bread crumbs and sea salt. Set aside.
2) In another bowl, prepare the buffalo coating by mixing the buffalo sauce and melted vegan butter. Set aside.
3) Dip the cauliflower florets in the buffalo coating, then dredge them in the panko mixture.
4) Place the cauliflower florets in the air fryer basket and air fry at 350° Fahrenheit (177° Celsius) for 17 minutes. There's no need to preheat the air fryer.
5) Shake the air fryer basket a few times to cook evenly.
6) Serve with the vegan mayonnaise as dipping sauce.

64. Air-Fried Ranch Kale Chips

Serving Size: 2

Calories: 150 per serving

Ingredients:
- ¼ tsp. salt
- 1 tbsp. nutritional yeast
- 2 tsp. vegan ranch seasoning
- 4 cups loosely-packed kale, rinsed and stems removed
- 2 tbsp. olive oil

Instructions:
1) Toss all ingredients in a mixing bowl. Make sure that the kale is coated with the oil and nutritional yeast.
2) Cook in an air fryer at 370° Fahrenheit (188° Celsius) for 5 minutes. Shake the fryer basket every 2 minutes. There is no need to preheat the air fryer.
3) Serve warm.

65. Texas Roadhouse Fried Pickles

Serving Size: 4

Calories: 78 per serving

Ingredients:

For the dip
- ¼ tsp. Cajun seasoning
- 1 tbsp. ketchup
- 1 tbsp. horseradish
- ¼ cup vegan mayonnaise

For the pickles
- 2 cups dill pickles, drained and sliced
- Salt to taste
- 1/8 tsp. cayenne pepper
- ¼ tsp. oregano
- 1 tsp. Cajun seasoning
- ¼ cup flour
- Oil for brushing

Instructions:

1) In a bowl, mix together all the ingredients for making the dip. Set aside.
2) In another bowl, mix flour with Cajun seasoning, basil, salt, pepper, and oregano.
3) Coat the pickles with the flour mixture. Brush with oil.
4) Preheat the air fryer to 392° Fahrenheit (200° Celsius).
5) Cook the pickles for 15 minutes or until the coating is golden brown.
6) Serve with the vegan mayonnaise dip.

66. Vidalia Onion Strings with Horseradish Aioli

Serving Size: 4

Calories: 255 per serving

Ingredients:

For the onion strings
- Salt and pepper to taste
- 1 ½ cup cornmeal
- 1 ¼ cup non-dairy milk
- 1 large Vidalia onion, sliced into rings
- Oil for brushing

For the aioli
- Salt and pepper to taste
- Juice of ½ lemon
- 2 tbsp. horseradish cream
- ½ cup vegan mayonnaise

Instructions:

1) In a large bowl, pour the non-dairy cream and add the onions. Separate the onion rings individually, using your fingers. Set aside.
2) In a shallow dish, transfer the cornmeal and add salt and pepper to taste.
3) Dredge the onion rings in the cornmeal mixture.
4) Brush with oil.
5) Cook in a preheated air fryer to 392° Fahrenheit (200° Celsius)) for 15 minutes until golden brown.

67. Baked Zucchini Fries

Serving Size: 3

Calories: 100 per serving

Ingredients:

- Salt and pepper to taste
- ¼ tsp. garlic powder
- Oil for brushing
- 2 tbsp. nutritional yeast
- ½ cup bread crumbs
- 1 cup non-dairy milk
- 3 medium-sized zucchini, sliced into sticks

Instructions:

1) In a small bowl, mix together non-dairy milk, salt, and pepper. Set aside.
2) In another bowl, combine the bread crumbs, nutritional yeast, and garlic powder. Mix well and set aside.
3) Dip the zucchini sticks into the wet mixture before you dredge it in the bread crumbs. Do this a few times.
4) Place the breaded zucchini at the bottom of the air fryer basket and brush cooking oil lightly.
5) Air fry for 20 minutes in a 392° Fahrenheit (200° Celsius) preheated air fryer or until golden brown.
6) Serve with any dipping sauce that you like.

68. Air-Fried Nuts

Serving Size: 4

Calories: 424 per serving

Ingredients:
- 2 cups of nuts of your choice
- A pinch of salt
- 1 tsp. olive oil

Instructions:
1) Preheat the air fryer to 320° Fahrenheit (160° Celsius) for 3 minutes.
2) Spread nuts in the fryer basket. Cook for 9 minutes and make sure to toss the nuts every 3 minutes.
3) Transfer the roasted nuts into a mixing bowl and add salt and oil.
4) Put the nuts back into the fryer, then cook for another 5 minutes.
5) Let cool before serving.

69. Air-Fried Banana Bread

Serving Size: 4 small loaves

Calories: 206 per loaf

Ingredients:

- ⅓ cup chopped pecans, toasted
- 1/8 tsp. baking powder
- ¼ tsp. baking soda
- ¼ tsp. salt
- ¼ tsp. ground nutmeg
- 1 tsp. ground cinnamon
- ¾ tsp. vanilla extract
- ¼ cup granulated sugar
- 2 tbsp. flaxseed meal mixed with 6 tbsp. water
- ¼ cup light brown sugar
- ½ very ripe banana, peeled and mashed
- ¾ cup all-purpose flour + more for dusting
- 4 tbsp. oil

Instructions:

1) Grease a small baking pan that can fit your air fryer. You can also use a ramekin if you don't have a small baking pan. Bake the banana bread by batch.
2) In a medium bowl, mix together ½ of the banana with oil and brown sugar. Add the flaxseed meal, granulated sugar, cinnamon, vanilla extract, and nutmeg. Add salt and mix well.
3) Add in the baking powder, baking soda, and flour. Fold until well combined. Add the pecans and mix well.
4) Place the batter on the greased pans or ramekins.
5) Preheat the air fryer to 320° Fahrenheit (160° Celsius) for 5 minutes.
6) Place the ramekins in the air fryer and bake for 20 - 25 minutes or until a toothpick inserted in the middle comes out clean.
7) Cook the other batches of the batter.

70. Air-Grilled Vegan Cheese Sandwich

Serving Size: 1

Calories: 114 per serving

Ingredients:
- A dollop of vegan butter
- ¼ cup shredded vegan cheese
- 2 slices whole meal soft bread

Instructions:
1) Preheat the air fryer to 356° Fahrenheit (180° Celsius) for 5 minutes.
2) Spread the cheese on the bread and cover with another slice of bread.
3) Place the sandwich on the fryer basket and add a dollop of butter on top.
4) Air fry for 3 - 5 minutes until the bread is brown on the sides.

71. Broccoli Hash Brown Cheese Cups

Serving Size: 6 large cups

Calories: 89 per cup

Ingredients:

- ¼ cup non-vegan milk
- ¼ cup vegan cheddar cheese, grated
- 2 tbsp. corn flour
- ½ block soft tofu, mashsed finely
- 3 tbsp. nutritional yeast
- ½ small head broccoli, florets broken into small pieces
- Salt and pepper to taste
- 2 tsp. olive oil
- 2 medium-sized potatoes, peeled and grated

Instructions:

1) Preheat the air fryer to 400° Fahrenheit (204° Celsius) for 5 minutes.
2) Place the grated potatoes in a kitchen towel and wring it to remove the excess liquid.
3) Place the dry potatoes in a mixing bowl and add olive oil. Add salt and pepper to taste. This will be your raw hash.
4) Divide the raw hash mix between six muffin molds and press to the bottom to create the crust. Air fry for 15 minutes.
5) Meanwhile, cook the broccoli florets in a microwave oven for 5 minutes until soft.
6) In a bowl, mix the tofu, nutritional yeast, milk, and corn flour.
7) Take the baked hash brown from the air fryer and add the cooked broccoli on top. Pour the tofu mixture into the cups.
8) Put the muffin pan back into the air fryer and cook for another 15 minutes.

72. Crispy Homemade Veggie Nuggets

Serving Size: 20 small nuggets

Calories: 65 per nugget

Ingredients:
- ½ tsp. black pepper
- ½ tsp. salt
- 2 cloves garlic, chopped finely
- 1 tbsp. olive oil
- 1 serrano pepper, seeded and chopped finely
- 1 stalk broccoli, blanched and grated
- 1 golden beet, blanched and grated
- 2 small potatoes, blanched and grated
- 1 parsnip, blanched and grated
- 3 medium-sized carrots, blanched and grated
- 1 cup non-dairy milk
- 2 cups bread crumbs

Instructions:
1) In a mixing bowl, mix all grated vegetables and add garlic and olive oil. Season with black pepper and salt. Mix until well combined.
2) Create 1-inch logs out of the vegetable mixture and set aside. Freeze for an hour inside the fridge.
3) Preheat the air fryer to 400° Fahrenheit (204° Celsius) for 5 minutes.
4) Take the veggie logs from the fridge and dredge each piece with milk first, then the bread crumbs.
5) Arrange individual nuggets in the air fryer and make sure that there is enough space for the air to flow within the basket. Air fry for 15 to 20 minutes or until golden brown.

73. Banana-Nutella Spring Rolls

Serving Size: 12 spring rolls

Calories: 93 per spring roll

Ingredients:
- 1 cup Nutella spread
- 1 package spring roll wrappers
- 6 whole bananas, peeled and halved

Instructions:
1) Preheat the air fryer to 375° Fahrenheit (190° Celsius) for five minutes.
2) Unwrap spring roll wrappers. Place a banana half at the center of the wrapper. Put 1 tablespoon of Nutella spread on the side of the banana half.
3) Roll the spring roll wrappers and tuck the corners to seal the contents. Use water to seal the edges.
4) Place in the air fryer and cook for 15 minutes or until the spring roll wrappers are crispy and brown.

74. Mashed Potato Tater Tots

Serving Size: 1

Calories: 191 per serving

Ingredients:
- Salt and pepper to taste
- 1 tsp. onion, minced
- 1 tsp. oil
- 1 red potato

Instructions:
1) Chop the potatoes finely and place in a pot of boiling water. Cook for 5 minutes or until soft.
2) Place the potatoes in a bowl and mash. Add in the rest of the ingredients.
3) Set the air fryer to 379° Fahrenheit (192 Celsius) and preheat for 5 minutes.
4) Form the potatoes into tater tot logs and air fry for 8 minutes. Shake the fryer basket then cook for another 5 minutes.
5) Serve with ketchup.

75. Cheese Spinach Balls

Serving Size: 4

Calories: 123 per serving

Ingredients:

- 1 ½ cups spinach, finely shredded and blanched
- ½ cup bread crumbs
- 3 tbsp. nutritional yeast
- 1 tsp. red chili flakes
- 1 onion, chopped finely
- 3 tbsp. brown rice flour
- 2 cloves garlic, grated
- Salt and pepper to taste
- Oil for brushing

Instructions:

1) Mix all ingredients in a mixing bowl. Season with salt and pepper to taste. Toss until well combined.
2) Form small balls and coat lightly with oil.
3) Preheat the air fryer to 392° Fahrenheit (200° Celsius) for 5 minutes.
4) Place the balls in the air fryer basket and cook for 15 minutes.
5) Serve hot with tomato sauce or ketchup.

76. Oil-Free French Fries

Serving Size: 6

Calories: 80 per serving

Ingredients:
- Packaged French fries (154 grams)

Instructions:
1) Preheat the air fryer to 392° Fahrenheit (200° Celsius) for 5 minutes.
2) Place the French fries into the air fryer and cook for 15 to 20 minutes.
3) Serve with ketchup.

77. Sweet Corn Fritters

Serving Size: 25 small fritters

Calories: 24 per fritter

Ingredients:

- 1 tbsp. coriander leaves, chopped
- 4 spring onions, sliced
- ½ red capsicum, diced
- 4 corn cobs, kernels removed
- ½ cup non-dairy milk
- 1 tbsp. flaxseed meal mixed with 3 tbsp. water
- 1 tsp. sea salt
- 1 tbsp. sugar
- 1 tsp. paprika
- 1 tsp. baking powder
- 1 cup all-purpose flour
- 2 tbsp. nutritional yeast

Instructions:

1) Sift the flour, paprika, and baking powder in a bowl. Add the sugar and salt.
2) In a separate bowl, mix together the flaxseed meal and non-dairy milk.
3) Add the wet ingredients to the dry ingredients. Mix the batter to remove the lumps. Set aside.
4) In a bowl, mix the corn kernels, capsicum coriander, and spring onions.
5) Mix the batter into the vegetable mixture.
6) Preheat the air fryer to 392° Fahrenheit (200° Celsius) for 5 minutes.
7) Form balls and cook the fritters for 20 to 25 minutes until brown.

78. Three Sister Squash

Serving Size: 6

Calories: 173 per serving

Ingredients:

- Salt and pepper to taste
- 1 tsp. paprika
- ½ cup fresh parsley, minced
- 1 ½ cups cooked brown rice
- 2 cups broccoli florets, diced
- 2 cups corn kernels
- 3 cups cooked black beans
- 2 serrano chilies, minced
- 1 cup red onion, diced
- 3 acorn squash
- 3 cloves garlic, minced
- 1 tbsp. olive oil

Instructions:

1) Preheat the air fryer to 392° Fahrenheit (200° Celsius) for 5 minutes.
2) In a small bowl, combine the olive oil and garlic. Set aside.
3) Prepare the squash by cutting it in half vertically. Scoop out the seeds and brush inside the squash with the garlic oil. Roast the squash in the air fryer for 35 minutes.
4) Heat the oil in a skillet under medium-low heat. Sauté the onion and chili for two minutes.
5) Add the garlic, corn, beans, and broccoli. Mix in the rice and cook for 5 minutes.
6) Stir in the paprika, parsley, salt, and pepper.
7) Remove the squash from the air fryer and put the filling in the middle of the squash.

79. Onion Rings

Serving Size: 6 to 8

Calories: 113 per serving

Ingredients:
- Salt and pepper to taste
- 2 cups bread crumbs
- 1 tbsp. baking powder
- ½ cup cornstarch
- 1 cup flour
- 1 cup water
- 2 onions, peeled and sliced into rings

Instructions:
1) In a bowl, mix together cornstarch, flour, baking powder, and salt.
2) Place the onion rings one at a time on the flour mixture to coat. Set aside.
3) Once the onion rings are coated with the flour mixture, add water, and pepper. Whisk until smooth.
4) Dredge the floured onion rings in the batter, then into the bread crumbs.
5) Cook in a preheated air fryer at 392° Fahrenheit (200° Celsius) for 20 to 25 minutes or until golden brown.

80. Portobello Mushroom Bacon

Serving Size: 4

Calories: 81 per serving

Ingredients:
- Salt and pepper to taste
- 2 oz. liquid smoke
- ¼ cup maple syrup
- 1 large Portobello mushroom, washed then sliced
- 1 tbsp. coconut oil

Instructions:
1) Marinate the mushroom slices with the liquid smoke and maple syrup for one hour. Season with salt and pepper.
2) Preheat the air fryer to 392° Fahrenheit (200° Celsius) for 5 minutes.
3) Brush the marinated mushroom with oil and cook in the air fryer for 30 minutes until the mushroom is crispy.

Mexican Recipes

81. Quinoa Taco Meat

Serving Size: 3

Calories: 84 per serving

Ingredients:

- ¾ cup water
- 1 cup vegetable broth
- 1 cup tri-color quinoa
- 1 tbsp. olive oil
- ½ tsp. salt
- ½ tsp. black pepper
- ½ tsp. garlic powder
- 2 tsp. ground chili
- 2 tsp. cumin powder
- 1 tbsp. nutritional yeast
- ½ cup prepared salsa

Instructions:

1) In a saucepan over medium heat, toast the quinoa for 5 minutes.
2) Add the water and vegetable broth and bring to a boil over medium-high heat. After 5 minutes, reduce the heat to low and cook for 15 to 25 minutes or until the quinoa has absorbed the liquid. Fluff the quinoa with a fork and let it rest with the lid slightly open.
3) Preheat the air fryer to 375° Fahrenheit (190° Celsius) for 5 minutes.
4) Once cooled, transfer the quinoa to a large bowl and add the remaining ingredients.
5) Toss inside the air fryer basket and bake for 35 minutes.
6) Shake the basket every 5 minutes to cook the quinoa taco meat evenly.
7) Serve with nachos or tacos.

82. Wonton Quesadillas

Serving Size: 12 small quesadillas

Calories: 102 per quesadilla

Ingredients:

- 2 tbsp. cilantro leaves, chopped
- 1 tsp. vegetable oil
- 12 gyoza or wonton wrappers
- 1 cup vegan cheese
- 1/8 tsp. cayenne pepper, ground
- ¼ tsp. coriander, ground
- ¼ tsp. cumin, ground
- ¼ cup canned refried beans

Instructions:

1) In a bowl, combine the spices and canned refried beans. Add in the vegan cheese and mix to incorporate all ingredients.
2) Divide the mixture evenly for the wonton wrappers. Spread the mixture and fold the wrapper. Do not seal.
3) Preheat the air fryer to 375° Fahrenheit (190° Celsius) for 5 minutes.
4) Place the wonton quesadillas in the fryer basket and cook for 5 to 8 minutes or until the wonton turns golden brown.
5) Garnish with cilantro leaves.

83. Corn Tortilla Chips

Serving Size: 10

Calories: 54 per serving

Ingredients:
- Salt to taste
- 1 tbsp. olive oil
- 8 corn tortillas

Instructions:
1) Preheat the air fryer to 392° Fahrenheit (200° Celsius) for 5 minutes.
2) Cut the corn tortillas into smaller triangles.
3) Brush each triangle with olive oil.
4) Place the tortilla pieces in the air fryer basket and cook for 3 minutes.
5) Sprinkle with salt.

84. Patatas Bravas

Serving Size: 4

Calories: 284 per serving

Ingredients:

- Salt and pepper to taste
- 1 tsp. rosemary
- 1 tsp. oregano
- 2 tsp. thyme
- 2 tsp. coriander
- 1 tsp. chili powder
- 1 tsp. paprika
- 2 tbsp. olive oil
- 1 tbsp. red wine vinegar
- 1 tomato, diced thinly
- 1 cup tomato sauce
- 1 small onion, peeled and diced
- 3 large potatoes, peeled and sliced into chips

Instructions:

1) Coat the potato chips with olive oil and place them in the air fryer basket and cook for 15 minutes at 362° Fahrenheit (183° Celsius).
2) Meanwhile, mix the rest of the ingredients in a mixing bowl.
3) Take the potatoes out once they are done and place the tomato mixture in the air fryer. Cook for 8 minutes.
4) Arrange the potatoes in a bowl and pour the tomato sauce over the chips. Serve warm.

85. Air-Fried Mushroom Taquitos

Serving Size: 12 taquitos

Calories: 77 per taquito

Ingredients:

- 1 cup vegan cheese, shredded
- 2 tbsp. canola oil
- ½ tsp. chili powder
- Salt and pepper to taste
- 1 tsp. garlic, minced
- 1 onion, chopped
- 1 ½ cup oyster mushroom, shredded
- 12 corn tortillas

Instructions:

1) Preheat the air fryer to 425° Fahrenheit (218° Celsius) for 5 minutes.
2) In a skillet, heat the canola oil and sauté the garlic and onion until wilted. Add the mushrooms. Season with salt and pepper to taste and cook for 3 to 5 minutes. Set aside.
3) Place the filling in the center of the corn tortilla and fold over the tortilla over the filling. Roll tightly just as you would when making a spring roll.
4) Place the taquitos in the air fryer and cook for 12 minutes or until golden brown.

86. Spicy Mexican Baby Potatoes

Serving Size: 4

Calories: 65 per serving

Ingredients:

For the baby potatoes

- 2 tbsp. oil
- 1 tsp. cilantro leaves for garnish
- 2 tsp. lime juice
- 2 cups baby potatoes

For Mexican seasoning

- ¼ tsp. cayenne pepper
- 1 tsp. paprika powder
- ½ tsp. garlic powder
- 1 tsp. oregano
- 1 tsp. cumin powder
- 1 tsp. salt

Instructions:

1) Prepare the Mexican seasoning by mixing all ingredients. Set aside.
2) Prepare the potatoes by parboiling them in boiling water until slightly tender. Once boiled, slice the potatoes into halves.
3) Mix the potatoes and the Mexican seasoning. Toss lightly until coated.
4) Preheat the air fryer to 392° Fahrenheit (200° Celsius) and cook for 8 to 12 minutes or until the potatoes are crisp and golden.

87. Air-Fried Nachos

Serving Size: 12 small nachos

Calories: 54 per nacho

Ingredients:
- 1 tablespoon canola oil
- ½ tsp. chili powder
- Salt to taste
- 1 cup all-purpose flour
- ½ cup fresh sweet corn, ground into a fine paste

Instructions:
1) In a bowl, mix all the ingredients together and knead to make a stiff dough.
2) Preheat the air fryer to 356° Fahrenheit (180° Celsius) for 3 minutes.
3) Dust the dough with a little bit of flour and roll into thin sheet.
4) Cut into desired shapes. Place the nachos in the air fryer basket and fry for 7 minutes.
5) Serve with salsa.

88. Mexican Plantain Chips

Serving Size: 4

Calories: 105 per serving

Ingredients:
- Four raw plantain bananas, peeled and sliced thinly
- Salt and pepper to taste
- Oil for brushing

Instructions:
1) In a mixing bowl, combine the bananas and oil. Toss to coat the bananas with oil.
2) Preheat the air fryer to 356° Fahrenheit (180° Celsius) for 5 minutes.
3) Transfer the bananas into the air fryer basket and cook for 10 minutes.

89. Air-Fried Vegan Refried Beans

Serving Size: 8

Calories: 197 per serving

Ingredients:
- 1 tsp. salt
- ½ tsp. black pepper
- 1 tsp. ground cumin
- 2 tsp. Mexican oregano
- 4 cups water
- 4 cups vegetable broth
- 2 cups pinto beans, rinsed
- 1 jalapeno, minced
- 4 cloves garlic, minced
- 1 onion, chopped

Instructions:
1) In a skillet, sauté the garlic, onion, and jalapeno. Add the rinsed beans, water, and veggie broth. Add the seasoning. Cook for 15 minutes.
2) Transfer the beans into another container and place the container in a preheated air fryer at 392° Fahrenheit (200° Celsius).
3) Continue cooking in the air fryer for another 15 minutes or until the liquid has reduced.
4) Mash the beans and serve with nachos.

90. Mexican Zucchini Burrito Boats

Serving Size: 8-10 boats

Calories: 337 per boat

Ingredients:
- 1 cup vegan cheese, shredded
- Salt to taste
- ½ cup fresh cilantro, chopped
- 1 tsp. chili powder
- 2 tsp. cumin
- 1 tbsp. olive oil
- 1 jalapeno pepper, cored and diced
- ½ cup corn kernels
- ½ cup onions, diced
- 1 red bell pepper, cored and diced
- 1 cup prepared salsa
- 1 cup cooked brown rice
- 1 15-oz. can black beans, drained and rinsed
- 4 large zucchini, halved and sliced to fit the air fryer

Instructions:
1) Hollow out the center of each zucchini and brush with olive oil. Place skin-side down.
2) In a large skillet, heat a tablespoon of olive oil and sauté the onions and peppers. Cook for 2 - 3 minutes. Add the rice, beans, and corn. Mix in the salsa, chili, and cumin. Mix everything then set aside. Add cilantro and salt to the filling.
3) Preheat the air fryer to 400° Fahrenheit (204° Celsius).
4) Spoon the filling into the hollowed-out center of the zucchini.
5) Place in the air fryer and cook for 25 minutes.

91. Creamy Bean Taquitos

Serving Size: 15 taquitos

Calories: 29 per taquito

Ingredients:

- 15 6-inch corn tortillas
- ⅓ tsp. salt
- ⅓ tsp. pepper
- ⅓ tsp. garlic powder
- 3 dashes of hot sauce
- 2 green onions, chopped
- 4 oz. can green chilies, diced
- 15 oz. can black beans
- 4 oz. vegan cream cheese

Instructions:

1) In a mixing bowl, combine all ingredients except the corn tortillas.
2) Place the filling in the middle of the corn tortillas and fold the edges to secure the filling.
3) Preheat the air fryer to 400° Fahrenheit (204° Celsius).
4) Cook for 15 minutes or until the bean taquitos are golden brown.

92. Deep Fried Guacamole

Serving Size: 6

Calories: 35 per serving

Ingredients:
- 2 cups tortilla chips, crushed
- 1 lemon wedge, juiced
- A dash of white pepper
- ¼ tsp. coarse salt
- ½ small onion, chopped
- 1 clove garlic, minced
- 1 plum tomato, diced
- 2 ripe avocados, peeled and seeded

Instructions:
1) In a bowl, mix together the tomatoes, avocadoes, garlic, and onion. Mash using a fork and season with salt and pepper to taste. Add the lemon juice. Mix again until well combined. Chill.
2) Once chilled, make small balls and roll the balls into the crushed tortilla chips.
3) Preheat the air fryer to 400° Fahrenheit (204° Celsius) for 5 minutes.
4) Cook for 15 minutes.

93. Baked Black Bean and Sweet Potatoes Flauta

Serving Size: 9

Calories: 150 per serving

Ingredients:

- Vegan sour cream for dipping
- Parsley for garnish
- Olive oil for brushing
- Salt and pepper to taste
- 1 tbsp. salsa
- 4 oz. of grated vegan cheese
- 2 oz. cashew cream cheese
- ¼ tsp. cayenne pepper
- ½ tsp. cumin
- ½ tsp. dried cilantro
- ½ tsp. garlic powder
- ½ tsp. chili powder
- ¼ cup diced red onion
- 1 small sweet potato, boiled and fluffed
- 1 cup corn
- 1 cup black beans
- 9 corn tortillas

Instructions:

1) In a mixing bowl, combine the minced peppers, corn, onion, and black beans. Add the garlic powder, cumin, chili powder, cilantro, salsa, and cayenne pepper.
2) Add the sweet potatoes to the spice mixture and add salt, as well as additional seasoning to taste. Add the rest of the ingredients except the corn tortillas.
3) Add the filling to the center of the corn tortillas. Do not fold the edges; secure the flautas with a toothpick.
4) Preheat the air fryer to 400° Fahrenheit (204° Celsius) for 5 minutes.
5) Cook the flautas for 15 minutes until crisp.

94. Crispy-Baked Tofu Tacos with Lime-Cilantro Slaw

Serving Size: 4

Calories: 167 per serving

Ingredients:

- Hot sauce for dipping
- 8 corn tortillas, heated and charred
- 1 tbsp. + 1 tbsp. olive oil
- 1 lime, juiced
- ¼ cup chopped cilantro
- 3 green onions, sliced
- 4 cups shredded cabbage
- ½ tsp. cumin
- 4 tbsp. nutritional yeast
- 2 tbsp. soy sauce
- 1 16oz. block of extra firm tofu, drained and cubed

Instructions:

1) In a mixing bowl, combine the nutritional yeast, soy sauce, 1 tbsp. olive oil, and cumin. Season with salt and pepper. Add the tofu cubes and toss to coat. Marinate 30 minutes.
2) Preheat the air fryer to 400° Fahrenheit (204° Celsius) for 5 minutes.
3) Place the marinated tofu cubes in the air fryer basket and bake for 30 minutes, flipping every 5 - 10 minutes.
4) While the tofu is in the air fryer, make the slaw by mixing the cabbage, cilantro, and green onions in a bowl. In another smaller bowl, combine the rest of the olive oil and lime juice. Season with salt and pepper. Add the dressing to the slaw and toss to combine.
5) Once the tofu is cooked, place the tofu and slaw in the tortilla.
6) Serve with hot sauce.

95. Baked Vegan Chimichangas

Serving Size: 3

Calories: 195 per serving

Ingredients:

- Salsa of your choice
- 1 cup lettuce, shredded
- 1 cup refried beans
- 4 burrito-size flour tortillas
- ¼ cup adobo sauce
- 1 cup shredded seitan or 1 large Portobello mushroom
- A pinch of salt
- 1 nopales cactus or large zucchini, trimmed and cut into ¾-inch cubes

Instructions:

1) Heat a skillet over medium flame and sauté the cactus paddle. Season with salt and cook for 8 minutes. Set aside.
2) In the same skillet, toss the Portobello mushroom and add the adobo sauce.
3) Assemble the tortillas by spreading ¼ cup refried beans, Portobello mushroom, shredded lettuce, and sautéed cactus on one size.
4) Roll the tortilla and close halfway. Fold the top and bottom inward to close the wrapper.
5) Brush with oil lightly.
6) Preheat the air fryer to 400° Fahrenheit (204° Celsius) for 5 minutes.
7) Air fry the chimichangas for 15 minutes until golden brown.
8) Serve with salsa.

96. Spicy Braised Tofu Tostadas

Serving Size: 3

Calories: 225 per serving

Ingredients:

For tostadas
- 2 tbsp. grape seed oil
- 6 white corn tortillas

For toppings
- Cilantro for garnish
- 1 red onion, diced
- Hot sauce for dipping
- Salsa of your choice
- Guacamole of your choice

For tofu filling
- ½ cup red salsa
- 1 cup vegetable broth
- 1 chipotle pepper in adobo sauce
- 1 tsp. garlic powder
- 1 ½ tsp. ground cumin
- 1 ½ tsp. chili powder
- 10 oz. extra firm tofu, drained and crumbled
- ¼ tsp. salt and black pepper
- ½ white onion, diced
- 5 cloves garlic, minced
- 2 tbsp. grape seed oil

Instructions:

1) Heat a large skillet over medium heat. Add grapeseed oil and sauté onion, garlic, and bell pepper. Season with salt and pepper. Cook for another 4 minutes until the vegetables are slightly brown.
2) Add the tofu and cook for another 5 minutes. Stir constantly to avoid burning the bottom. Add the cumin, chili powder, and garlic powder.
3) Mix in the chipotle pepper, salsa, and broth. Reduce the heat to low and simmer for 15 minutes.
4) Meanwhile, preheat the air fryer to 356° Fahrenheit (180° Celsius). Brush the tortilla with oil and air fry for 8 minutes.
5) Assemble the tostadas by arranging the braised tofu and toppings in the middle of the corn tortillas.

97. Lentil Picadillo

Serving Size: 4

Calories: 123 per serving

Ingredients:

- 1 large carrot, diced
- 2 medium potatoes, peeled and diced
- ½ tsp. black pepper
- ½ tsp. salt
- ½ tsp. cumin
- 1 jalapeno, finely chopped
- 3 cloves garlic, minced
- ½ large white onion, chopped
- 2 medium tomatoes, chopped
- 3 cups water
- 8 oz. brown lentils, cooked
- Vegan mozzarella cheese

Instructions:

1) In a skillet, heat the oil over medium heat. Sauté the onions for 5 minutes or until soft.
2) Add the garlic and jalapeno and cook for a minute more. Add the cooked lentils and stir for 1 minute.
3) Add the tomatoes and cumin, then season with salt and pepper.
4) Mix in the diced carrots and potatoes.
5) Place the picadillo in ramekins and top with vegan mozzarella cheese.
6) Preheat the air fryer to 356° Fahrenheit (180° Celsius) and place inside the ramekins.
7) Continue to cook the picadillo in the air fryer for 10 minutes.
8) Garnish with lime and cilantro.
9) Serve with warm tortillas.

98. Vegan Chiles Rellenos

Serving Size: 4

Calories: 278 per serving

Ingredients:

For the batter
- 1 ½ cups soda water
- 1 tsp. salt
- 1 cup cornstarch
- 1 cup all-purpose flour

For the chilies
- ½ onion, peeled and chopped
- 2 cloves garlic, chopped
- 3 tomatoes, chopped
- 10 oz. vegan cheese
- 4 poblano peppers, roasted and peeled

Instructions:

1) Cut the poblano chilies vertically in half. Fill them with your favorite vegan cheese. Close the chili by placing the other half on top. Secure with a toothpick. Set aside.
2) Make the batter by combining all the batter ingredients. Set aside.
3) Make the sauce by blending the tomatoes, onion, and garlic until smooth. Set aside.
4) In a medium sauce pan, add the tomato sauce and simmer until the sauce begins to thicken. Season with salt and pepper.
5) Dredge the chilies in the batter. Remove the excess batter, then set aside.
6) Preheat the air fryer to 356° Fahrenheit (180° Celsius).
7) Air fry the chilies for 15 minutes.
8) Serve with the tomato sauce.

99. Air-Fried Vegan Fajitas

Serving Size: 2

Calories: 125 per serving

Ingredients:

For the fajita seasoning
- A dash of red pepper flakes
- ¼ tsp. cumin
- ¼ tsp. garlic powder
- ¼ tsp. onion powder
- ½ tsp. paprika
- 1 tsp. sugar
- 1 tsp. salt
- ½ tsp. black pepper
- 1 tbsp. chili powder

For the fajitas
- 1 red onion, sliced
- 1 each of red, green, orange, and yellow bell pepper, sliced
- 2 large Portobello mushrooms, sliced

Instructions:

1) In a bowl, mix together all of the fajita seasoning ingredients, then set aside.
2) In another bowl, mix the fajita ingredients.
3) Add the prepared seasoning.
4) Preheat the air fryer to 356° Fahrenheit (180° Celsius) for 5 minutes.
5) Cook for at least 15 to 20 minutes.
6) Serve with vegan sour cream, guacamole, or tortillas.

100. Crispy Black Bean Tacos

Serving Size: 12 tortillas

Calories: 199 per tortilla

Ingredients:

For avocado-lime sauce
- 2 tbsp. water
- 1 tbsp. sugar
- A pinch of salt
- 1 tsp. taco seasoning
- ⅓ cup olive oil
- 1 jalapeno, seeded
- 3 limes, juiced
- ½ bunch cilantro
- 2 avocados

For the black beans
- 12 corn tortillas
- ¾ cup vegan cheese
- 3 cups Mexican black beans, cooked and drained
- Salt and pepper to taste

Instructions:
1) In a bowl, mix together beans and vegan cheese.
2) Preheat the air fryer to 356° Fahrenheit (180° Celsius) for 5 minutes.
3) Cook the beans and cheese in the air fryer for 15 to 20 minutes.
4) Once the beans are cooked, place the tortillas in the air fryer and heat for 8 minutes.
5) Prepare the avocado-lime sauce by combining all ingredients except the avocado.
6) Assemble the tacos by placing the bean mixture in the center of the taco. Add avocado and drizzle with the lime sauce.
7) Fold the tortillas and serve with salsa.

101. Mexican Quinoa Stuffed Peppers

Serving Size: 4

Calories: 325 per serving

Ingredients:
- 1 tsp. chili powder
- 1 tsp. smoked paprika
- 1 ½ tsp. cumin
- 2 tbsp. nutritional yeast
- ⅔ cup salsa
- 2 green onions, chopped
- 1 cup corn
- 15 oz. can black beans
- ¾ cup dry quinoa
- 4 large bell peppers

Instructions:
1) Cook the quinoa according to package instructions.
2) Prepare the bell peppers by cutting them in half and removing the seeds and ribs.
3) In a large mixing bowl, add the cooked quinoa and the rest of the ingredients except the bell peppers. Mix until well combined and season with salt and pepper to taste.
4) Preheat the air fryer to 350° Fahrenheit (176° Celsius) for 5 minutes.
5) Fill the bell peppers with the quinoa filling and cook in the air fryer for 20 to 25 minutes.
6) Serve with any toppings that you like.

Conclusion

Staying healthy all the time is one of the more challenging tasks of life. We try different diets, healthier food, better workout routines, and so on. It requires a lot of time, effort, and motivation to become fit, but perhaps we can start small by incorporating healthier choices into our lives.

One of the simplest changes that we can make to become healthier is to stay away from food that is prepared using unhealthy cooking methods. It's a small change that can have a huge positive impact on your health. Air frying is definitely a better alternative than deep frying, especially if combined with the vegan diet. This combination ensures that you are getting the necessary nutrients in your body through food that was prepared the right way!

Thousands of hours have been spent on scientific research about the vegan diet, and you will hear about the success stories everywhere. However, you will not experience the benefits first-hand if you don't try it yourself.

Hopefully this book has helped you get closer to a healthier lifestyle, and has made your cooking experience more fun.

And Please...

If you'd like more quality diet books at this low price, we'd really appreciate a review on Amazon. The number of reviews a book has is directly related to how it sells, so even leaving a very short review will help make it possible for us to continue to do what we do.

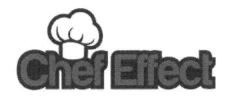

Other Books By Chef Effect

To find out more about other books that we have written, please visit our Author Central Page by going to the webpage below or scanning the QR code.

https://goo.gl/5IUi6k

Made in the USA
Middletown, DE
23 November 2017